Oxford Specialist Handbooks in Cardiology

Nuclear Cardiology

Nikant Sabharwal
Specialist Registrar in Cardiology
John Radcliffe Hospital
Oxford, UK

Chee Yee Loong
Specialist Registrar in Cardiology
Hammersmith Hospital
London, UK

and

Andrew Kelion
Consultant Cardiologist
Royal Brompton & Harefield NHS Trust
Harefield, UK

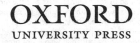

OXFORD
UNIVERSITY PRESS

OXFORD
UNIVERSITY PRESS

Great Clarendon Street, Oxford OX2 6DP

Oxford University Press is a department of the University of Oxford.
It furthers the University's objective of excellence in research, scholarship,
and education by publishing worldwide in

Oxford New York

Auckland Cape Town Dar es Salaam Hong Kong Karachi
Kuala Lumpur Madrid Melbourne Mexico City Nairobi
New Delhi Shanghai Taipei Toronto

With offices in

Argentina Austria Brazil Chile Czech Republic France Greece
Guatemala Hungary Italy Japan Poland Portugal Singapore
South Korea Switzerland Thailand Turkey Ukraine Vietnam

Oxford is a registered trade mark of Oxford University Press
in the UK and in certain other countries

Published in the United States
by Oxford University Press Inc., New York

© Oxford University Press, 2008

The moral rights of the authors have been asserted
Database right Oxford University Press (maker)

First published 2008

British Library Cataloguing in Publication Data
Data available

Library of Congress Cataloging in Publication Data
Data available

Typeset by Newgen Imaging Systems (P) Ltd., Chennai, India
Printed in Italy
on acid-free paper by
Legoprint S.p.A

ISBN 978–0–19–920644–5 (flexicover: alk.paper)

10 9 8 7 6 5 4 3 2 1

Foreword

Drs Sabharwal, Loong, and Kelion have provided a superb and up-to-date guide to the basic concepts and clinical applications of nuclear cardiology. The handbook is very practically organized in condensed chapters that cover all issues in an elegant manner. Nuclear cardiology has become an important component in the daily, clinical management of patients with cardiac disease, and this book provides a good introduction to physicians who are not familiar with nuclear cardiology, but at the same time offers an excellent update for clinicians who have been involved with nuclear cardiology previously. The authors have created a perfect balance between physics, equipment, and tracers on the one hand and clinical applications on the other hand. The text is clear and the chapters are illustrated with practical case examples.

The handbook can be divided into three major components: the first part deals with the basics of nuclear cardiology, ranging from radiation physics to imaging equipment, including collimators and gamma cameras.

The second and largest part of this handbook is dedicated to SPECT myocardial perfusion imaging. Indeed myocardial perfusion imaging with SPECT, has developed over the past decades into an extremely useful technique in the daily management of patients with suspected or known coronary artery disease. SPECT perfusion imaging has an excellent diagnostic accuracy to detect coronary artery disease, in combination with either physical exercise or pharmacological stress. Strong prognostic information is also provided with SPECT perfusion imaging; it is well known that a normal stress-rest myocardial perfusion study carries an excellent long-term prognosis. Alternatively, the risk for cardiovascular events increases in parallel to the extent of perfusion abnormalities on stress-rest perfusion imaging. Accordingly, SPECT perfusion imaging has been implemented in the daily clinical management and risk stratification of patients with known or suspected coronary artery disease.

All aspects of SPECT myocardial perfusion imaging are discussed in this superb handbook, including practical issues such as stress testing, available tracers, and image interpretation. An elegant chapter is included on the clinical use of SPECT perfusion imaging, covering the diagnostic and prognostic value of the technique.

The third part of the book includes chapters on novel tracers and positron emission tomography (PET). One chapter concerns the use of new iodine-123 labelled tracers, including MIBG and BMIPP. Neuronal imaging with MIBG is a promising technique, particularly useful for risk stratification in patients with heart failure. BMIPP is a fatty acid analogue that permits for ischemic memory imaging; in patients who encountered an episode of ischemia, perfusion may have normalized, but oxidative metabolism can still be reduced, and this can be imaged with BMIPP.

These novel iodine-123 labelled SPECT tracers reflect specific patho-physiological processes that could not be imaged with SPECT before. PET is the most sophisticated technique in nuclear cardiology. Extensive information on PET instrumentation and radiopharmaceuticals is provided in a chapter dedicated to PET imaging. The clinical applications of this technique are discussed in detail, with special emphasis on viability imaging with F18-fluorodeoxyglucose.

This handbook will be an extremely valuable guide to the use of nuclear cardiology for physicians involved in the contemporary practice of clinical cardiology.

Jeroen J Bax
Professor of Cardiology
Leiden University Medical Center
The Netherlands

Preface

We hope that clinicians will find this a readable, practical, and self-contained guide to nuclear cardiology, covering both technical and clinical aspects. No book can be a substitute for hands-on experience in a high-volume centre, but we have tried to provide a foundation of essential knowledge that should be common to physicians of any background training in the subspecialty.

Nuclear cardiology requires a combination of technical and clinical expertise which many medical practitioners find it hard to acquire in training. Nuclear physicians and radiologists are well versed in radiation protection and imaging technologies, but often have limited understanding of the subtleties of current patient management in cardiology. They may fail to appreciate the impact of the wording of their reports on the minds of referring cardiologists. Conversely, cardiologists have a good understanding of stress testing and the clinical implications of a given scan appearance, but often lack a good grounding in the technical issues. They can often struggle to satisfy national legal requirements for running a service, and may overlook technical factors that make a particular scan appearance unreliable.

These deficiencies are mirrored in the available texts. Books specifically about nuclear cardiology usually provide excellent detail on the clinical aspects of the subspecialty, but readers are directed elsewhere for in-depth coverage of radiation physics and imaging technology. Books on general nuclear medicine provide detailed technical information on radionuclide imaging in general, but often gloss over the more clinical aspects of cardiac imaging in the limited space available. Few books provide a practical step-by-step guide to nuclear cardiology procedures, despite the standardization of many aspects. We hope that we have gone some way towards rectifying this.

NS
CL
AK

August 2007

Contents

Contents

Detailed contents

Symbols and abbreviations

AC	attenuation correction
ADP	adenosine diphosphate
ALARA	as low as reasonably achievable
ALS	advanced life support
AMP	adenosine monophosphate
ARSAC	Administration of Radioactive Substances Advisory Committee
ATP	adenosine triphosphate
Bckgnd	background counts
Bq	becquerel
CABG	coronary artery bypass graft surgery
CASS	Coronary Artery Surgery Study
Ci	curie
CMR	cardiac magnetic resonance
CT	computed tomography
CTA	computed tomography angiography
DEFRA	Department for the Environment, Food and Rural Affairs
DIAD	Detection of Ischaemia in Asymptomatic Diabetics
DH	Department of Health
EA	Environment Agency
ECG	electrocardiogram
EDC	end-diastolic counts within LV ROI
EF	ejection fraction
EMPIRE	Economics of Myocardial Perfusion Imaging in Europe
END	Economics of Noninvasive Diagnosis
FRASE	Emergency Room Assessment of Sestamibi for Evaluation
ERNV	equilibrium radionuclide ventriculography
ESC	end-systolic counts within LV ROI
FPRNV	first-pass radionuclide ventriculography
GTN	glyceryl trinitrate
H/M ratio	heart-to-mediastinum ratio
HCM	hypertrophic cardiomyopathy
HR	heart rate
HSA	human serum albumin
HSE	Health and Safety Executive
ICD	implantable cardioverter-defibrillator
ICRP	International Commission for Radiation Protection
INSPIRE	adenosine sestamibi SPECT post-infarction evaluation
IRMER	Ionising Radiation (Medical Exposures) Regulations 2000

IRR99	Ionising Radiations Regulations 1999
LAD	left anterior descending
LAO	left anterior oblique
LBBB	left bundle branch block
LCx	left circumflex
LV	left ventricle/ventricular
MARS	Medicines (Administration of Radioactive Substances) Regulations 1978/1995
MBq	megabecquerels
mCi	millicuries
MIRD	medical internal radiation dose
MPS	myocardial perfusion scintigraphy
MUGA	multi-gated acquisition
NSTEMI/UAP	non-STEMI and unstable angina pectoris
OM	obtuse marginal
PCI	percutaneous coronary intervention
PDA	posterior descending artery
PET	positron emission tomography
PHA	pulse height analyzer
PMTs	photomultiplier tubes
QC	quality control
RAO	right anterior oblique
RCA	right coronary artery
RNV	radionuclide ventriculography
ROI	region of interest
RPA	Radiation Protection Advisor
RPS	Radiation Protection Supervisor
RSA93	Radioactive Substances Act 1993
RV	right ventricle
SAM	S-adenosyl methionine
SC	stroke counts
SDS	summed difference score
SNM	Society of Nuclear Medicine
SPECT	single photon emission computed tomography
SRS	summed rest score
SSS	summed stress score
STEMI	ST-elevation myocardial infarction
Sv	sievert
TAC	time-activity curve
TID	transient ischaemic dilatation
TIMI	thrombolysis in myocardial infarction
W_R	radiation weighting factor
W_T	tissue weighting factor
μ_{linear}	linear attenuation coefficient

Chapter 1

Introduction to nuclear cardiology

Introduction

The cardiologist of the early twenty-first century takes for granted the wide range of imaging modalities at his/her disposal, but it was not always so. At the beginning of the 1970s, invasive cardiac catheterization was the only reliable cardiac imaging technique. Subsequently, nuclear cardiology investigations led the way in the non-invasive assessment of cardiac disease. Some of the principles underlying these investigations [e.g. electrocardiogram (ECG)-triggered gating] have also been of great importance in the development of other imaging modalities.

Equilibrium radionuclide ventriculography was the first reliable non-invasive method of quantifying left ventricular function, and has been widely performed since the mid-1970s. In combination with exercise it also provided the first stress-rest imaging technique for assessing inducible ischaemia in patients with known or suspected coronary disease. Myocardial perfusion scintigraphy was slower to develop initially, but has now become by far the dominant nuclear cardiology investigation.

Important milestones

General nuclear medicine

- 1927. Blumgart and Weiss used ^{214}Bi to measure pulmonary circulation time from a venous site in one arm to an arterial site in the other: the first 'first-pass' study.
- 1950. Cassen developed a sensitive directional γ-ray detector for imaging the distribution of ^{131}I in the thyroid: the first rectilinear scanner.
- 1957. Hal Anger developed the gamma camera which bears his name and which revolutionized radionuclide imaging; the first camera came onto the market in 1961.
- 1960. Richards developed the ^{99}Mo/^{99m}Tc generator system; this became commercially available in 1965, allowing ^{99m}Tc to become the dominant radionuclide used in imaging.

Left ventricular function

- 1971. Strauss and colleagues pioneered equilibrium radionuclide ventriculography: the blood pool was labelled with ^{99m}Tc-albumin, and gating was used to acquire separate diastolic and systolic images; ejection fraction was calculated geometrically from left ventricular regions of interest.
- 1972. The background-corrected counts-based approach was introduced to measure left ventricular ejection fraction in the left anterior oblique projection.
- 1974. Acquisition became possible throughout the cardiac cycle, with generation of time-activity curves, making equilibrium radionuclide ventriculography more practical.
- 1976. Borer demonstrated the value of exercise equilibrium radionuclide ventriculography as an investigation for coronary disease.

Myocardial perfusion

- 1964. Carr injected intracoronary ^{131}Cs during cardiac catheterization to image myocardial perfusion.
- 1970. Kawana proposed ^{199}Tl as a myocardial perfusion tracer.
- 1973. Zaret used intravenous ^{43}K to demonstrate exercise-induced regional reductions in myocardial perfusion in coronary disease.
- 1974. Lebowitz developed ^{201}Tl, which had better imaging characteristics than ^{43}K; ^{201}Tl became commercially available from 1976.
- 1978. Gould introduced pharmacological stress with dipyridamole.
- 1979. Jasczak developed the first single photon emission computed tomography (SPECT) gamma camera; the first camera came onto the market in 1984.
- 1984. ^{99m}Tc-sestamibi was described, and was approved for clinical use in the USA in 1990; ^{99m}Tc-labelled tracers became increasingly popular during the 1990s.
- 1991. Gated SPECT was introduced, and became increasingly practical with the introduction of multi-headed gamma cameras in the 1990s.

Relation to other imaging modalities

Introduction

In the mid 1970s, scintigraphic techniques were the only methods available for imaging the heart non-invasively. The last 30 years have seen major developments in imaging technology, and nuclear cardiology now competes with echocardiography, magnetic resonance imaging, and X-ray computed tomography (CT) in the investigation of cardiology patients. In some parts of the developed World, most notably in North America, nuclear cardiology (particularly myocardial perfusion scintigraphy) is recognized as a mature subspecialty, underpinned by an extensive literature. It has become firmly embedded in the management of large numbers of patients. In other parts of the World, for example in the UK, it has failed to become a mainstream investigation in most centres, often for medicopolitical rather than clinical reasons. In such countries there is a danger that newer and more fashionable techniques, which demonstrate similar aspects of cardiac physiology, will become widely established before their clinical and cost-effectiveness have been properly demonstrated.

Left ventricular function

Radionuclide ventriculography has been largely replaced by echocardiography in the everyday assessment of left ventricular function, and appropriately so. Gated SPECT provides an accurate assessment of left ventricular function in the setting of myocardial perfusion scintigraphy, but is not normally used as a stand-alone technique. Echocardiography is quick, widely available, and free of ionizing radiation. It may be argued that the ejection fraction provided by the radionuclide methods is more accurate and reproducible, but this is unimportant in the majority of cases where it is only necessary to know whether the left ventricle is normal or mildly/moderately/severely impaired.

Where accurate quantification *is* important, cardiac magnetic resonance (CMR) imaging now represents an important challenge to the radionuclide techniques as it appears to be more reproducible. However, CMR is expensive and not widely available, and its superiority is more relevant to research rather than clinical applications. Radionuclide ventriculography continues to have a niche role, for example in the serial assessment of patients undergoing chemotherapy.

Functional imaging in known or suspected coronary artery disease

Echocardiography and CMR offer alternatives to myocardial perfusion scintigraphy in the assessment of patients with suspected or known coronary disease:
- Echocardiography:
  - Stress echo (wall motion).
  - Myocardial contrast echo (perfusion).
- CMR:
  - Stress CMR (wall motion).
  - Perfusion CMR.

With the exception of stress echo, the evidence base underpinning these techniques is limited. However it is likely that in expert hands they provide more-or-less equivalent clinical information to perfusion scintigraphy. Moreover, they do not involve exposure to ionizing radiation, which may be an advantage in young low-risk patients.

The attractions of myocardial perfusion scintigraphy are primarily practical:
- Ability to deliver high volume service: a single dedicated cardiac gamma camera can study well over 2000 patients per year, with little requirement for hands-on medical input except in reporting (cf. stress echo).
- Applicable to all patients:
  - Imaging possible in all but most morbidly obese patients (due to weight limitations on imaging table), for whom cardiac catheterization is similarly impossible.
  - No difficulties with imaging windows (cf. echo).
  - Most cameras suitable for claustrophobic patients (cf. CMR).
  - No problems for those with pacemakers or other metal implants (cf. CMR).
- Operator independent: published evidence of good agreement between observers in reporting.
- Published evidence of cost-effectiveness:
  - Diagnostic strategies that involve perfusion scintigraphy are cheaper than those that do not, with no difference in clinical outcome.
  - Myocardial perfusion scintigraphy delivered at high volume is no more expensive than stress echocardiography, and certainly cheaper than CMR.

Challenge of multislice X-ray CT

Recently, multislice (currently 64-slice) X-ray CT has established itself as a realistic non-invasive alternative to invasive coronary angiography. Its role in relation to perfusion scintigraphy is still being defined, but a number of points are already clear:
- The two techniques are not interchangeable: perfusion scintigraphy is a functional assessment, whilst CT provides anatomical information about plaque burden (coronary calcium scoring) and stenoses (CT coronary angiography).
- The relative value of the two types of information will vary between patients, and in some individuals both may be helpful in providing a reliable assessment and avoiding unnecessary cardiac catheterization (hence the development of SPECT/CT cameras).
- CT angiography (CTA) is most reliable when it is normal, whilst perfusion scintigraphy is most valuable in intermediate risk patients: CTA may be most appropriate in low-risk patients.

Radiation physics, biology, and protection

Atoms and nuclei

Atom

An atom is the smallest particle of matter exhibiting the characteristic chemical properties of an element. It consists of a positively charged nucleus, orbited by an equivalent number of negatively charged electrons (if in the neutral or un-ionized state).

Nucleus

An atomic nucleus consists of two types of particle called *nucleons*:
- *Protons*: positive charge, equal and opposite to that of an electron.
- *Neutrons*: neutral charge.

A *nuclide* is a defined type of nucleus, characterized by:
- *Mass number*, A : total number of nucleons (protons and neutrons).
- *Atomic number*, Z : number of protons, defining chemical element of atom to which nuclide belongs.

In conventional notation, a nuclide, X, is represented as $^A_Z X$: for example, $^{14}_6 C$ is a nuclide containing 14 nucleons in total, of which 6 are protons and $14 - 6 = 8$ are neutrons. From the periodic table of elements (see Fig. 2.1), the element with atomic number 6 is carbon, hence 'C'. Given that an element is uniquely defined by its atomic number, the notation for a nuclide can be further shortened to $^A X$ (e.g. ^{14}C = carbon-14).

Nuclides can be grouped into families:
- Isotopes have the same number of protons and are the same element (e.g. $^{201}_{81}Tl$ and $^{201}_{81}Tl$).
- Isobars have the same mass number, A (e.g. $^{99}_{42}Mo$ and $^{99}_{43}Tc$).
- Isotones have the same number of neutrons (e.g. $^3_1 H$ and $^4_2 He$).
- In addition to a ground state, nuclides can exist at different energy levels or excited states: isomers. A relatively stable isomer with a half-life $\geq 1\mu s$ is termed 'metastable' (e.g. ^{99m}Tc).

Electrons

Electrons are much lighter than nucleons, and carry a negative charge which is equal and opposite to that of a proton.

Electrons are arranged in characteristic shells at increasing distance from the nucleus (K, L, M, etc.), each of which can hold a maximum number (2, 8, 18, etc.). Under normal circumstances, inner shells must be filled before electrons can occupy outer shells. The chemical properties of a given element are largely determined by the number of outer shell valence electrons in its atoms which are available to form chemical bonds. The removal or addition of electrons from/to an atom leaves it positively or negatively charged (ionized).

Whenever an electron is removed from an inner shell, its place must be taken by an outer shell electron. The difference in binding energy between the two shells is released as a photon of electromagnetic radiation, or by the freeing of an outer shell (Auger) electron. If the energy of the photon is >100eV it is termed an X-ray, and its energy is characteristic for a particular element.

1	2	3	4	5	6	7	8	9	10	11	12	13	14	15	16	17	18
1 H Hydrogen 1.00794																	2 He Helium 4.003
3 Li Lithium 6.941	4 Be Beryllium 9.012182											5 B Boron 10.811	6 C Carbon 12.0107	7 N Nitrogen 14.00674	8 O Oxygen 15.9994	9 F Fluorine 18.9984032	10 Ne Neon 20.1797
11 Na Sodium 22.989770	12 Mg Magnesium 24.3050											13 Al Aluminium 26.981538	14 Si Silicon 28.0855	15 P Phosphorus 30.973761	16 S Sulfur 32.066	17 Cl Chlorine 35.4527	18 Ar Argon 39.948
19 K Potassium 39.0983	20 Ca Calcium 40.078	21 Sc Scandium 44.955910	22 Ti Titanium 47.867	23 V Vanadium 50.941	24 Cr Chromium 51.9961	25 Mn Manganese 54.938049	26 Fe Iron 55.845	27 Co Cobalt 58.933200	28 Ni Nickel 58.6934	29 Cu Copper 63.546	30 Zn Zinc 65.39	31 Ga Gallium 69.723	32 Ge Germanium 72.61	33 As Arsenic 74.92160	34 Se Selenium 78.96	35 Br Bromine 79.904	36 Kr Krypton 83.80
37 Rb Rubidium 85.4678	38 Sr Strontium 87.62	39 Y Yttrium 88.90585	40 Zr Zirconium 91.224	41 Nb Niobium 92.90638	42 Mo Molybdenum 95.94	43 Tc Technetium (98)	44 Ru Ruthenium 101.07	45 Rh Rhodium 102.90550	46 Pd Palladium 106.42	47 Ag Silver 107.8682	48 Cd Cadmium 112.411	49 In Indium 114.818	50 Sn Tin 118.710	51 Sb Antimony 121.760	52 Te Tellurium 127.60	53 I Iodine 126.90447	54 Xe Xenon 131.29
55 Cs Caesium 132.90545	56 Ba Barium 137.327	57 La Lanthanum 138.9055	72 Hf Hafnium 178.49	73 Ta Tantalum 180.9479	74 W Tungsten 183.84	75 Re Rhenium 186.207	76 Os Osmium 190.23	77 Ir Iridium 192.217	78 Pt Platinum 195.078	79 Au Gold 196.96655	80 Hg Mercury 200.59	81 Tl Thallium 204.3833	82 Pb Lead 207.2	83 Bi Bismuth 208.98038	84 Po Polonium (209)	85 At Astatine (210)	86 Rn Radon (222)
87 Fr Francium (223)	88 Ra Radium (226)	89 Ac Actinium (227)	104 Rf Rutherfordium (261)	105 Db Dubnium (262)	106 Sg Seaborgium (263)	107 Bh Bohrium (262)	108 Hs Hassium (265)	109 Mt Meitnerium (266)	110 (269)	111 (272)	112 (277)	113	114 (277)				

58 Ce Cerium 140.116	59 Pr Praseodymium 140.90765	60 Nd Neodymium 144.24	61 Pm Promethium (145)	62 Sm Samarium 150.36	63 Eu Europium 151.964	64 Gd Gadolinium 157.25	65 Tb Terbium 158.92534	66 Dy Dysprosium 162.50	67 Ho Holmium 164.93032	68 Er Erbium 167.26	69 Tm Thulium 168.93421	70 Yb Ytterbium 173.04	71 Lu Lutetium 174.967
90 Th Thorium 232.0381	91 Pa Protactinium 231.03588	92 U Uranium 238.0289	93 Np Neptunium (237)	94 Pu Plutonium (244)	95 Am Americium (243)	96 Cm Curium (247)	97 Bk Berkelium (247)	98 Cf Californium (251)	99 Es Einsteinium (252)	100 Fm Fermium (257)	101 Md Mendelevium (258)	102 No Nobelium (259)	103 Lr Lawrencium (262)

Fig. 2.1 The periodic table of the elements.

Radioactive decay

Of the approximately 1800 known nuclides, only about 300 are stable. Stable nuclides are characterized by approximately equal numbers of protons and neutrons, or by an excess of neutrons for A >100. An unbalanced ('parent') nuclide is unstable, and attempts to achieve stability by radioactive decay into a 'daughter' nuclide with the release of energy as electromagnetic or particulate radiation. Such unstable nuclides are termed *radionuclides*. A daughter nuclide may itself be unstable, and may decay further via a series of steps until a stable nuclide is produced. Radioactive decay processes are not affected by environmental conditions or chemical binding.

There are three modes of radioactive decay:
- Alpha (α).
- Beta (β).
- Gamma (γ).

In all cases, the following are conserved:
- Energy (sum of mass energy by $E = mc^2$, kinetic energy, and electromagnetic energy).
- Mass number (total number of nucleons).
- Electric charge.

α decay

The nucleus emits an α-particle, which is a helium nucleus ($^4_2$He) consisting of two protons and two neutrons without orbital electrons:

$$\text{for example, } ^{226}_{88}\text{Ra} \rightarrow {}^{222}_{86}\text{Rn} + {}^4_2\text{He}$$

β decay

A neutron changes into a proton or *vice versa*. The daughter nuclide is an isobar of its parent (same mass number, but different atomic number, i.e. element). There are three types of β decay:

β^- *decay*

A neutron changes into a proton with the release of a negatively charged β-particle (an electron) and an anti-neutrino (required to conserve energy, but of no biological relevance):

$$n \rightarrow p^+ + e^- + \mu$$

for example, decay of molybdenum-99 to technetium-99m in a technetium generator:

$$^{99}_{42}\text{Mo} \rightarrow {}^{99m}_{43}\text{Tc} + e^- + \mu$$

β^+ *decay*

A proton changes into a neutron with the release of a positively charged β-particle (an anti-electron or positron) and a neutrino (required to conserve energy, but of no biological relevance):

$$p^+ \rightarrow n + e^+ + \nu$$

for example, decay of fluorine-18 used to label ^{18}FDG for positron emission tomography (PET) imaging:

$$^{18}_{9}F \rightarrow \ ^{18}_{8}O + e^+ + \nu$$

The positron is an antimatter particle which travels less than a millimetre before undergoing an annihilation reaction on meeting a free electron. Charge is neutralized, and all the mass energy is converted into a pair of 511keV photons travelling in opposite directions.

Electron capture

An orbital electron, usually from the innermost K shell, is captured by the nucleus and combines with a proton to form a neutron:

$$p^+ + e^- \rightarrow n + \nu$$

for example, decay of thallium-201 used in myocardial perfusion scintigraphy:

$$^{201}_{81}Tl \ + e^- \rightarrow \ ^{201}_{80}Hg + \nu$$

The net result for the nuclide is similar to β^+ decay. The vacancy created in the inner electron shell is filled by an outer shell electron, with emission of a characteristic X-ray (or Auger electron).

γ decay

Following decay, a nuclide can exist in an excited state due to the absorption of energy. When the nuclide decays to a lower energy isomer, this energy can be released in one of two ways:

- Emission of a high-energy γ photon, indistinguishable from an X-ray photon but for its origin.
- Internal conversion, where an inner shell (conversion) electron is ejected; subsequent filling of the vacancy leads to emission of a characteristic X-ray photon.

A given isomer can undergo either process with characteristic probability.

Statistics of radioactive decay

Units of radioactivity

The radioactivity (activity) of a sample of radionuclide is the number of decays per unit time. In SI units, 1 becquerel (Bq) is equivalent to 1 decay per second. The older unit, the curie (Ci), is a much larger unit equivalent to 3.7×10^{10} decays per second (the activity of a 1g sample of ^{226}Ra). In nuclear medicine, radiopharmaceutical doses are typically measured in megabecquerels (MBq) or millicuries (mCi), with 1mCi equivalent to 37MBq.

Exponential law of decay

The atoms of a given radionuclide have a characteristic probability of decay over a given time, the decay constant (λ). The rate of decay of a sample of N_t atoms is

$$-dN_t/dt = \lambda N_t$$

which predicts the exponential law of decay:

$$N_t = N_0.e^{-\lambda t}$$

where N_0 is the number of atoms at baseline, and N_t the number remaining at time t. The same exponential decay applies to the radioactivity of a sample.

In everyday practice, the physical half-life of a radionuclide ($T_{1/2}$), the time taken for half of a sample to decay, is a more convenient parameter than the decay constant. It is related to the decay constant as follows:

$$T_{1/2} = 0.693/\lambda$$

For simple calculations, the exponential law of decay conveniently simplifies to

$$N_t = N_0 \times (1/2)^{\text{number of half-lives}} \text{ (see Fig. 2.2)}.$$

Physical, biological, and effective half-lives

In nuclear medicine, the removal of radioactivity from a patient is as much dependent on the biological properties of the radiopharmaceutical as it is on the physical half-life of the radionuclide. The *biological* half-life is the time taken for metabolism and excretion to eliminate half of a radiopharmaceutical dose. The *effective* half-life is the time taken to eliminate half of the radioactivity, and is related to both the physical and biological half-lives:

$$1/T_{1/2 \text{ effective}} = 1/T_{1/2 \text{ physical}} + 1/T_{1/2 \text{ biological}}$$

The effective half-life is therefore always less than or equal to the shorter of the physical or biological half-life.

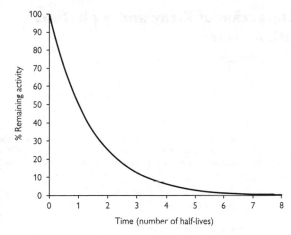

Fig. 2.2 Remaining activity of a sample of radionuclide as a function of the number of half-lives elapsed.

Interaction of X-ray and γ photons with matter

Linear attenuation coefficient

As high-energy photons pass through a material, they may be absorbed or scattered. The proportion of incident photons transmitted is an exponential function of the thickness of the material (x) and its *linear attenuation coefficient* (μ_{linear}):

$$N_x/N_0 = e^{-\mu_{linear} x}$$

The linear attenuation coefficient is related to photon energy and the physical properties of the material. The *half-value layer* of a material is the thickness which attenuates half of the incident photons, and equals

$0.693/\mu_{linear}$

For everyday calculations,

$$N_x/N_0 = (\tfrac{1}{2})^{\text{number of half-value layers}}$$

Photon interactions with matter

High-energy photons interact with matter in three ways:
- Photoelectric effect.
  - Photon completely absorbed by atom, all energy transferred to orbital electron which is ejected.
  - Atom is left ionized.
  - If ejected electron is from inner shell, characteristic X-ray or Auger electron also produced.
- Compton scatter.
  - Photon transfers only part of its energy to orbital electron, usually in outer shell, which is ejected.
  - Atom is left ionized.
  - Scattered lower energy photon emerges.
- Electron–positron pair production.
  - Does not occur at photon energies <1.02MeV, so not relevant in nuclear medicine.

The likelihood of both the photoelectric effect and Compton scatter:
- Decreases with increasing photon energy
- Increases with increasing atomic number of the material

but with very different functions. Thus one or other phenomenon tends to be dominant for photons of a given energy travelling through a particular medium (see Fig. 2.3). For photons of energy 50–300keV:

- Body tissue   Compton scatter
- Lead   Photoelectric effect
- Sodium iodine   Photoelectric effect

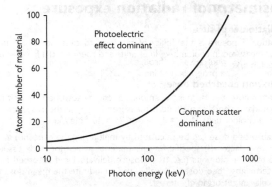

Fig. 2.3 Graph of photon energy versus atomic number of absorber, to show regions of predominantly photoelectric effect versus Compton scatter. NB ^{99m}Tc photon energy 140keV, atomic number: lead 82, iodine (gamma camera crystal) 53, oxygen (tissue) 8.

Dosimetry of radiation exposure

Radiation exposure

Radiation exposure is the ability of radiation to cause ionization in air, and is measured in coulomb/kg in SI units and roentgen (R) in older units (1 coulomb/kg = 3876R).

Radiation absorbed dose

Radiation absorbed dose is the amount of energy absorbed per unit mass of material or body tissue, and is measured in gray in the SI system (Gy) and rad in older units ($1Gy = 1J/kg$ or 6.24×10^{12} MeV/kg).

The absorbed dose can be calculated by multiplying the exposure at that point by a factor (f) specific for the material, which for body tissues is close to 1 for old units (i.e. 1R exposure delivers 1 rad absorbed dose). The term 'absorbed dose' is usually used to indicate the mean dose to a particular target organ of interest.

Equivalent dose

Equivalent absorbed doses of different types of radiation are not equally detrimental to biological systems. Equivalent dose weights the absorbed dose to allow for these differences, and is a better indicator of the potential harm to living tissue:

equivalent dose = absorbed dose × radiation weighting factor (W_R)

The SI unit is the sievert (Sv) and the older unit the rem. For the radiation encountered in nuclear medicine (X-ray and γ photons, electrons and positrons), W_R is equal to 1. α-particles and neutrons are much more damaging for a given absorbed dose, and have a correspondingly higher W_R of 10–20.

Just as different types of radiation have different biological effects for a given absorbed dose, so different tissues have different susceptibilities to damage. A *tissue-weighted radiation equivalent* dose can be calculated by multiplying the radiation equivalent dose by a tissue weighting factor (W_T; see Table 2.1). The *radiation effective* dose is then the sum of the tissue-weighted equivalent doses for all the exposed tissues, and is expressed in Sv or rem.

MIRD scheme

When a radiopharmaceutical is administered to a patient, it is impossible in practice to measure the dose to any specific organ. Calculations must be performed based on computer modelling of a standard patient. The scheme that is universally used is that developed by the Medical Internal Radiation Dose (MIRD) committee of the American Society of Nuclear Medicine (SNM); the software is called MIRDOS. The approach relies upon knowledge of:

• Decay scheme of radionuclide.
• Dynamics and distribution of radiopharmaceutical in patient.
• Fraction of energy emitted from each source organ that is absorbed by each target organ.

Table 2.1 Tissue weighting factor (W_T) and risk per sievert for different body tissues

Tissue	Probability of fatal cancer ($\times 10^{-2}$/Sv)	W_T
Gonads	0.10	0.20
Bone marrow	0.50	0.12
Colon	0.85	0.12
Lung	0.85	0.12
Stomach	1.10	0.12
Bladder	0.30	0.05
Breast	0.20	0.05
Liver	0.15	0.05
Oesophagus	0.30	0.05
Thyroid	0.08	0.05
Skin	0.02	0.01
Bone surface	0.05	0.01
Other	0.50	0.05
TOTAL	5.00	1.00

Biological effects of radiation exposure

Radiation exerts its effects on biological systems via energy deposition causing ionization. This can damage important biological molecules, such as DNA, directly. More commonly, damage is indirect due to the production of reactive free radicals (H· and OH·) from water molecules.

The effects of radiation in human can be divided into acute and late effects.

Acute effects

The acute effects of radiation are *deterministic* and conform to a *linear-threshold model*: that is, the severity of the effect is directly proportional to the radiation dose, but below a certain dose threshold no effect is seen. These threshold doses are generally much higher than are encountered in diagnostic nuclear cardiology (above 50mSv but typically 500mSv), and acute radiation effects such as damage to the bone marrow and gastrointestinal lining are not an issue either for patients or healthcare professionals.

Late effects

The late effects of radiation exposure are mainly *stochastic* and are assumed to conform to a *linear-no-threshold model*: that is, the probability of occurrence, but not the severity, increases linearly with dose but with no lower threshold. The most important and relevant late effects of radiation exposure are cancer induction and, to a much lesser extent, genetic damage. Thus although the risk of cancer induction is low at low doses, there is assumed to be no 'safe' level of exposure and all radiation must be regarded as potentially deleterious. This has led to the adoption of the ALARA principle in radiation protection: all exposures should be kept As Low As Reasonably Achievable, taking social and economic factors into account. It is worth noting that several recent lines of evidence have challenged the linear-no-threshold model, suggesting that radiation exposure at the levels encountered in diagnostic nuclear medicine may not be as harmful as predicted.

As a rule of thumb, radiation exposure at the levels encountered in nuclear cardiology are considered to confer an increase in the lifetime risk of fatal cancer of:

• 5×10^{-2} per Sv in the general population.
• 4×10^{-2} per Sv in people of working age.
• After a 10 year latency.
• Against a background risk of fatal cancer of 1 in 3.

Table 2.2 indicates the risks associated with tracer protocols used in myocardial perfusion scintigraphy.

Table 2.2 Risk of cancer induction associated with radiopharmaceutical protocols used in myocardial perfusion scintigraphy

Radiopharmaceutical	Protocol	Dose (MBq)	Effective dose equivalent (mSv)	Lifetime risk of fatal cancer
Thallium-201	Stress-redistribution	80	14	1 in 1429
	Stress-reinjection	120	21	1 in 952
^{99m}Tc-sestamibi	Two-day	800	8	1 in 2500
	One-day	1000	10	1 in 2000
^{99m}Tc-tetrofosmin	Two-day	800	6	1 in 3333
	One-day	1000	8	1 in 2667

Principles of radiation protection

Control of radiation is based on the recommendations of the International Commission for Radiation Protection (ICRP). In the UK, responsibility for enforcing the limits falls to the Department of Health (DH) and the Department for the Environment, Food and Rural Affairs (DEFRA).

The goals of radiation protection are to prevent the occurrence of clinically significant deterministic effects by adhering to dose limits that are well below the threshold levels, and to minimize the risk of stochastic effects by ensuring that all exposures are as low as reasonably achievable (ALARA). The three fundamental principles are:
- Justification.
- Optimization.
- Limitation.

Justification

The medical value of the exposure should be greater than the risk. In practice this means that a responsible practitioner must authorize each request for an investigation, or produce a clear list of appropriate indications for others to follow.

Female patients of childbearing age are a difficult group:
- Known pregnancy or breastfeeding: nuclear cardiology procedures generally deferred.
- Known not to be pregnant: obtain signed confirmation prior to proceeding with investigation.
- Pregnancy status uncertain: apply '28-day rule', that is, perform test only if within 28 days of the last menstrual period when any embryo would be at a pre-organogenesis stage (congenital abnormalities unlikely).

Optimization

Radiation exposure should be as low as reasonably achievable for both patients and staff, allowing for the constraints of working procedures (for staff) and the importance of obtaining diagnostic images (for patients).

Limitation

Legal annual dose limits are produced for workers and members of the public (see Table 2.3 for the UK). Staff likely to exceed 30% of any of the annual dose limits for workers are designated as 'classified workers'. They are subject to careful dose monitoring and regular medical surveillance, and their records are held centrally by the Health and Safety Executive (HSE) for 50 years after the last entry. It would be most unusual for professionals involved in diagnostic nuclear cardiology to require 'classified' status.

Table 2.3 Current UK effective dose limits

Public	1mSv per year
Designated worker	5mSv per year
Classified worker	20mSv per year, averaged over 5 years

Radiation protection of staff

Protection from external sources

The minimization of radiation exposure is achieved by three general principles:
- Time.
- Distance.
- Shielding.

Time

Radiation dose is directly proportional to the time of exposure. Thus tasks which involve working with radioactive sources (including injected patients) should be completed as quickly as possible, though always with due care.

Distance

The flux from a source of γ or X-rays is inversely proportional to the square of the distance from it. Thus doubling the distance of a source from the body reduces the radiation dose by a factor of 4.

In practice, distance is the most important way of reducing exposure:
- Handle unshielded radiopharmaceutical doses with forceps.
- Hold doses away from the body whenever possible.
- Ensure imaging rooms large enough to allow staff to work at a reasonable distance from injected patients.

Shielding

In nuclear medicine, it is necessary to be very close to the source of radiation when preparing, carrying, or injecting doses of radiopharmaceutical. Exposure can be reduced by the use of appropriate lead shielding, for example, lead glass shields for preparing doses, syringe-shields, and lead carrying boxes. Lead aprons are less effective in nuclear medicine than they are in diagnostic radiology, only reducing exposure from ^{99m}Tc and ^{201}Tl photons by 25–50%, and are generally not used.

Protection from internal exposure

Internal exposure occurs when radionuclides enter the body, and can be avoided by preventing their release into the environment, and blocking the portals of entry by inhalation, ingestion and absorption through the skin (intact or broken). In nuclear cardiology, high concentrations (MBq/ml) of radiopharmaceuticals are used, and small spills can result in significant contamination of personnel and the working environment. The main vector of internal exposure is probably contaminated hands, which will lead to skin absorption and ingestion. Therefore:
- Do not eat, drink, smoke, or apply cosmetics in areas where unsealed sources are used.
- Wear lab coat and protective gloves when handling potentially contaminated items; dispose of gloves immediately in appropriate bin.
- Wash hands regularly.

- Wear appropriate personal dose monitors (e.g. film badge).
- Keep work surfaces tidy and cover with absorbent pads in case of spillage.
- Survey work areas, hands, and clothing regularly for contamination using portable scintillation crystal monitor.

Procedure in the event of a spill

In general, the radiopharmaceuticals used in nuclear cardiology do not present a major hazard, but any spill must be taken seriously and dealt with appropriately. Appropriate advice should be taken from a medical physics expert.

Decontamination of people

- Take care not to spread activity.
- Remove contaminated clothing, place in bag, and store behind shielding.
- Wash hands repeatedly and carefully, using appropriate purpose-made solution if necessary.
- Shower and wash hair if appropriate.

Decontamination of room

- Take care not to spread activity.
- Wear plastic gloves and apron.
- Cover liquid with paper towels.
- Define contaminated area with monitor and mark.
- Scrub repeatedly with appropriate purpose-made solution.
- Monitor activity from time to time until reaches acceptable level (e.g. $<30Bq/cm^2$).
- Ensure all cleaning equipment is bagged and stored as radioactive waste.
- If contamination is major or widespread, probably best to vacate and seal room with warning notices until activity has decayed.

Production of radionuclides

The radionuclides used in nuclear medicine are artificial, and are available from one of three sources:
- Nuclear reactor.
  - Made by neutron capture or nuclear fission.
  - Typically decay by β^- emission, for example, molybdenum-99, the parent of technetium-99m.
- Industrial accelerator or cyclotron.
  - Made by acceleration of positive particles into a stable nuclide target.
  - Typically decay by β^+ emission or electron capture, for example, thallium-201 and iodine-123
- Generator.
  - Made by decay of relatively long-lived parent radionuclide into clinically useful daughter radionuclide with shorter half-life, for example, technetium-99m:

$$^{99}_{42}\text{Mo} \ (T_{1/2} \ 67 \ hours) \ \rightarrow \ ^{99m}_{43}\text{Tc} \ (T_{1/2} \ 6 \ hours) + e^- + \mu$$

The ^{99}Mo-^{99m}Tc generator

The ^{99}Mo-^{99m}Tc generator is in widespread use in radiopharmacies worldwide, providing ^{99m}Tc more or less 'on tap' (see Fig. 2.4). The parent radionuclide, ^{99}Mo in the form sodium molybdate, is adsorbed on top of alumina in a glass column. When the generator is eluted with normal saline, the ^{99m}Tc dissolves as sodium pertechnetate ($NaTcO_4$), whilst the ^{99}Mo is retained. Maximal allowable levels are set for the amount of ^{99}Mo and alumina which can be detected in the eluate.

In a radionuclide generator, the long half-life parent is continuously decaying into the daughter, which is itself decaying with shorter half-life. An equilibrium is established where there is a fixed ratio between the amounts of parent and daughter, and a maximum yield is available from the generator. The available daughter activity then decays with the half-life of the parent. If the generator is eluted, it takes approximately 4 half-lives of the daughter radionuclide for equilibrium to be re-established, that is, 24 hours for a ^{99}Mo-^{99m}Tc generator. Repeat elution of the generator within 24 hours will yield less than the maximal obtainable activity (50% at 6 hours, 75% at 12 hours, 88% at 18 hours, 94% at 24 hours).

^{99m}Tc-pertechnetate from a generator can be used to reconstitute a range of radiopharmaceuticals provided in vials by the manufacturer (e.g. sestamibi or tetrofosmin). Each vial can provide multiple patient doses.

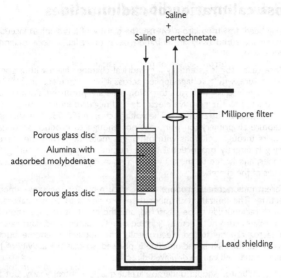

Fig. 2.4 Simplified diagram of a ^{99}Mo-^{99m}Tc generator.

Dose calibration of radionuclides

Having been drawn up into a syringe, the activity of a radiopharmaceutical must be measured using an ionization detector called a dose calibrator (see Fig. 2.5).

A dose calibrator is essentially a cylindrical chamber filled with argon at high pressure, with a voltage applied across it between electrodes. When γ or X-rays interact with gas atoms, ion pairs are produced. Positive ions are attracted to the negative electrode and negative ions to the positive electrode, and a current flows. The voltage chosen (50–250V) is sufficient to capture all primary ion pairs, but not enough to produce secondary ion pairs through collisions with other gas molecules. Thus the current flowing is directly proportional to the number of photons entering the chamber, and hence to the activity of a source placed in the well along the axis of the chamber.

Different radionuclides produce different currents for the same amount of activity. The ionization chamber therefore needs to be pre-calibrated for each radionuclide to be measured, and the constant of proportionality which relates current to activity (in MBq or mCi) determined. This calibration factor can be stored electronically and applied when the button appropriate for a given radionuclide is pressed, so that the activity of the sample in the well can be displayed directly.

A dose calibrator should undergo careful quality control yearly, but for more regular assurance the measured activity of a long-lived ^{137}Cs source of known activity can be assessed.

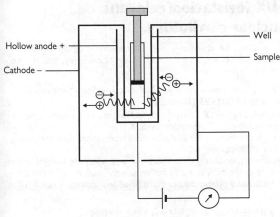

Fig. 2.5 Basic design of a dose calibrator (see text).

Key UK legislation relevant to nuclear cardiology

In most countries, the practice of nuclear medicine is tightly regulated. In the UK, a number of important pieces of legislation apply, and an overview of these is given below.

Medicines (Administration of Radioactive Substances) Regulations 1978/1995 (MARS)

- Administered by the DH through the Administration of Radioactive Substances Advisory Committee (ARSAC).
- All work is the responsibility of a medical practitioner who holds an ARSAC certificate.
- ARSAC certificate is only issued to those with adequate training and experience in the clinical use of radioactive substances and radiation protection, and if proper support is in place (equipment, medical physics).

Ionizing Radiations Regulations 1999 (IRR99)

- Administered by the HSE.
- Primarily concerned with protection of staff.
- Include requirements for informing HSE of use of radiation, prior risk assessment, local rules for radiation protection, Radiation Protection Advisor (RPA; a physicist), Radiation Protection Supervisor (RPS; usually a senior radiographer or technologist), source security, controlled areas, contingency plans.

Ionizing Radiation (Medical Exposures) Regulations 2000 (IRMER)

- Administered by the DH.
- Intended to ensure protection of patients and comforters or carers.
- Specific responsibilities placed on employer such as requirements for defined procedures and protocols.
- Definitions of various roles and their responsibilities: referrer, practitioner, operator, medical physics expert.

Radioactive Substances Act 1993 (RSA93)

- Regulated by the Environment Agency (EA).
- Intended to protect the environment from radioactive discharge.
- Regulates the holding and disposal of radioactive material.

The gamma camera

Crystals and collimators

Introduction

Nuclear cardiology imaging is performed on an Anger gamma camera. Its key component is a large flat circular or rectangular sodium iodide crystal, activated by non-radioactive thallium (NaI(Tl)). The side of the crystal facing the patient is covered with a lead collimator, whilst the side away from the patient is viewed by an array of photomultiplier tubes (PMTs).

NaI(Tl) crystal

Certain materials, known as scintillators, emit photons of visible light following interaction with γ photons via the photoelectric effect or Compton scatter. NaI(Tl) is overwhelmingly the most common scintillator used in gamma cameras, though others are more suitable for the detection of 511keV photons in positron emission tomography (PET) (e.g. bismuth germanate, lutetium oxyorthosilicate). Pure NaI is a poor scintillator, but the incorporation of a trace of thallium impurity increases the light produced by 10-fold or more. A single crystal is required or the light photons would be unable to travel out of it to be detected.

Light photons are emitted within 1mm of the causative interaction, with a total energy that is proportional to the energy given up by the γ photon. Approximately 1 light photon is emitted for every 30eV of γ-ray energy absorbed.

The crystal is fragile and hygroscopic, and requires hermetic sealing in an aluminium or stainless-steel envelope. It must also be protected from abrupt changes in temperature that can provoke mechanical stress and cracking.

Collimator

The collimator is to a gamma camera what a lens is to an optical camera. It allows only those X-rays or γ-rays which originate from a particular area of an organ to enter a selected area of the NaI(Tl) crystal, so maintaining spatial information.

In cardiac imaging, parallel-hole collimators are used. These consist of a lead disc penetrated by thousands of uniform parallel channels separated by thin septa. Only photons travelling perpendicular to the collimator can penetrate the channels and enter the crystal, whilst the remainder are absorbed by the lead septa (see Fig. 3.1).

A collimator typically allows only 1% of incident photons to reach the detector. Spatial resolution and sensitivity are related to the length and diameter of the channels: resolution increases whilst sensitivity falls with increasing length or decreasing diameter.
- 'High-resolution' collimators have relatively good resolution but poorer sensitivity and are commonly used for imaging [99m]Tc.
- 'High-sensitivity' collimators have high sensitivity but poorer resolution and are used in first-pass studies.
- 'All (general) purpose' collimators represent a balance between sensitivity and resolution and are often used with [201]Tl.

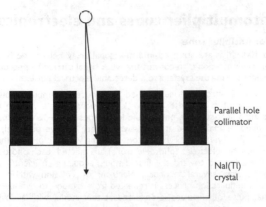

Parallel hole collimator

NaI(Tl) crystal

Fig. 3.1 Diagram of a parallel-hole collimator. Only photons travelling perpendicular to the face of the collimator can enter the crystal.

Photomultiplier tubes and electronics

Photomultiplier tube

Up to 100 PMTs are arranged in a hexagonal array behind the NaI(Tl) crystal. Their function is to convert the weak signal carried by photons of visible light leaving the crystal into a detectable electrical pulse.

A PMT is an electronic device designed to produce and amplify a pulse of electric current in response to a weak light signal. It is a vacuum tube containing a light-sensitive photocathode, a series of 10–12 metal plates called dynodes maintained at successively higher positive potential, and an anode. For every 3–10 light photons colliding with the photocathode, 1–3 low-energy electrons (photoelectrons) are ejected. Each photoelectron is accelerated toward the first dynode, acquiring sufficient kinetic energy to eject several secondary electrons on collision with it. The electron multiplication process is repeated from dynode to dynode until the final pulse of electrons is collected at the anode, with an overall multiplication factor of up to 10^7. The final pulse amplitude is proportional to the energy of the original light photons. Electron multiplication is also a sensitive function of the voltage differential between dynodes, so a stable voltage supply is vital.

Pulse arithmetic circuit

Light photons leaving the NaI(Tl) crystal activate nearby PMTs in a pattern related to the location of the originating scintillation event, with the largest electrical pulse being generated in the PMT closest to the event.

A microprocessor chip, called the pulse arithmetic circuit, combines the outputs from all PMTs in real-time to produce three voltage pulses: X, Y, and Z. The X and Y pulses represent the horizontal and vertical coordinates of the scintillation in the crystal, and hence (in the presence of a collimator) the position in the patient's body from which the γ photon originated. The Z pulse is proportional to the total light photon energy detected by the PMTs, and hence to the energy deposited by the original γ photon; for convenience it is expressed in keV.

Pulse height analyser

Using the Z pulses, a gamma camera can produce a histogram of photon energy against count rate which is characteristic for a particular radionuclide.

If the only γ-ray interaction were complete absorption via the photoelectric effect within the NaI(Tl) crystal, the energy spectrum would consist of one or more sharp 'photopeaks' corresponding to the energies of the emitted γ photons. In reality, not all scintillation events receive all of the original photon energy, either because energy has previously been lost via Compton scatter in the patient or detector, or because the scintillation event itself resulted from scatter rather than the photoelectric effect. The result is a Compton plateau in the energy spectrum, to the left of the photopeak (see Fig. 3.2 for ^{99m}Tc).

The spatial origin of scattered γ photons is uncertain, and they must therefore be eliminated from image acquisition. A pulse height analyser (PHA) allows selective counting of γ photons within a defined energy window around the photopeak, so eliminating scattered radiation: for example, for ^{99m}Tc a 20% energy window is typically used around the 140keV photopeak (126–154keV).

Correction circuitry

A modern gamma camera contains complex real-time circuitry for correction of linearity, PMT drift and energy. The aim is to optimize field uniformity and the correspondence between the location of scintillations in the NaI(Tl) crystal and their positions in the final image.

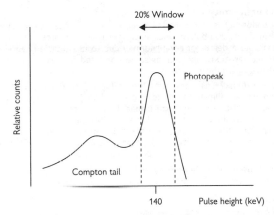

Fig. 3.2 Energy spectrum for ^{99m}Tc. Acquisition window between dotted lines represents 140keV ± 10%.

Gamma camera performance parameters and quality control (1)

Several important parameters characterize the performance of a gamma camera, and require regular monitoring as part of a programme of quality control (QC):
- Field uniformity.
- Spatial resolution.
- Sensitivity.
- High count rate performance.
- Energy resolution.

Field uniformity

Field uniformity is the ability of a gamma camera head to produce a uniform count distribution when imaging a uniform source. All cameras demonstrate a degree of non-uniformity due to unavoidable physical and electronic variations, and this must be corrected by careful 'tuning' to avoid imaging artefacts.

System (extrinsic) uniformity tests the uniformity of the entire imaging system with a collimator attached, and should be checked daily. An image is acquired of a sealed uniform planar flood source resting against the collimator, usually containing the long-lived isotope ^{57}Co. A visual check is made for inhomogeneities, which can be quantified and recorded as the integral non-uniformity (range of pixel count values) and differential non-uniformity (rate of change of pixel count values).

Intrinsic uniformity is checked by acquiring an image of a distant point source without a collimator. This is typically performed monthly.

Spatial resolution

Spatial resolution describes the ability of an imaging system to reproduce detail. The spatial resolution of a gamma camera is determined by the intrinsic resolution (i.e. the uncertainty in localizing a scintillation event within the crystal) and the collimator resolution.

Importantly, spatial resolution decreases with distance from the face of the collimator (see Fig. 3.3). Thus imaging should always be performed with the camera head as close as possible to the patient; this can be a challenge with single photon emission computed tomography (SPECT), where space must be allowed for the head(s) to travel around the patient.

Formal assessment of both intrinsic and system spatial resolutions involves imaging a line source, a thin tube filled with ^{99m}Tc. A line spread function, $L(x)$, is plotted as a bell-shaped graph of count rate against perpendicular distance from the source on either side, and spatial resolution can be expressed as the full width at half maximum (FWHM; see Fig. 3.4).

More straightforwardly, spatial resolution can be tested semiquantitatively with a parallel bar phantom to determine the smallest line spacing that can be identified. This may be done monthly.

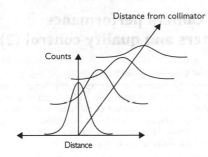

Fig. 3.3 Variation of line spread function (i.e. spatial resolution) with the distance from the face of a collimator.

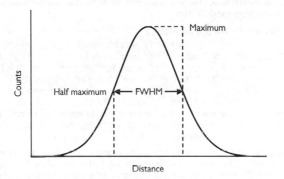

Fig. 3.4 Line spread function illustrating full width at half maximum (FWHM).

Gamma camera performance parameters and quality control (2)

Sensitivity

The sensitivity of a gamma camera is its ability to detect γ photons. It depends on both the intrinsic properties of the detector and on the collimator, and varies as the inverse square of the spatial resolution. Final image quality depends on the number of detected counts, and the extent to which radiopharmaceutical dosage or acquisition time can be increased is quite limited, so a pragmatic balance must always be sought between sensitivity and spatial resolution.

In practice, sensitivity can be quantified using a plane source containing a known activity of ^{99m}Tc, and expressed as the fraction of γ photons detected per unit time per unit area. More straightforwardly, the stability of system sensitivity can be checked crudely on a daily basis, at the same time as uniformity, by recording the time taken to acquire a given number of counts from the flood source.

High count rate performance

Following a scintillation event in the NaI(Tl) crystal, there is a dead time of 1–2µs during which other scintillations cannot be identified. If a second scintillation occurs during this period, the light photons will be added to the previous event. If both events are photoelectric interactions, the combined Z pulse exceeds the upper limit of the PHA energy window and both events will be incorrectly rejected. Therefore, whilst the observed count rate of a gamma camera is linearly related to activity at low activities, it saturates as activity increases. In nuclear cardiology this can be a problem for first-pass ventriculography.

Inadequate high count rate performance can also erode spatial resolution: if two sequential events involved Compton scatter, the sum of the two might fall within the energy window and be registered inappropriately as a single mispositioned scintillation event.

Energy resolution

Photopeaks calculated by the PHA are bell-shaped distributions as a result of statistical variations in both the number of light photons produced by each scintillation event, and the number of photoelectrons produced in the PMTs by each light photon. The narrower the photopeak the better the energy resolution of the detector, and this can be quantified as the FWHM. Good energy resolution allows a narrow acquisition window to collect a high proportion of the 'good' counts, optimizing spatial resolution and sensitivity.

Single photon emission computed tomography (SPECT)

Introduction to SPECT

Planar scintigraphic imaging represents a three-dimensional distribution of counts within a patient as a two-dimensional image. This results in a loss of contrast between the organ of interest and surrounding tissues due to activity in overlying and underlying structures.

Single photon emission computed tomography (SPECT) allows an organ to be imaged in three dimensions with enhanced contrast. Of particular relevance in nuclear cardiology, it also allows the heart to be reorientated relative to its own axes, and slices presented in standard orthogonal planes. Scintigraphic imaging is thereby rendered more accessible to cardiologists already familiar with echocardiography and other imaging modalities.

SPECT imaging involves the acquisition of a series of planar projections at different angles as the head(s) of the gamma camera orbit(s) the patient. Each projection requires fewer counts than would be acceptable for conventional planar imaging. A mathematical reconstruction method is then used to produce a set of transaxial sections through the patient.

Two methods of reconstruction can be used:
- Filtered back-projection.
- Iterative reconstruction.

The transaxial slices can then be reorientated to the axes of the heart.

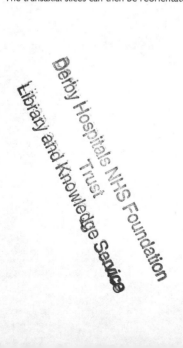

Specific issues of instrumentation, acquisition and processing

Camera options

Dual-headed versus single-headed

Dual-headed cameras are preferable to single-headed cameras for cardiac SPECT. By positioning the heads at 90° to each other, one head can be used to acquire the first 90° of a 180° orbit whilst the second simultaneously acquires the second 90°. Thus total acquisition time is halved, reducing the likelihood of significant patient motion and increasing patient throughput.

Dedicated cardiac camera versus general purpose camera

Dedicated cardiac gamma cameras are available with small heads fixed at 90° to each other. Image quality is equivalent to that of general purpose dual-headed cameras. Dedicated cardiac cameras offer two important advantages:

- Small size: can be installed in a relatively small room.
- Low cost: typically 40–60% that of general purpose cameras.

Cardiac cameras may play an important role in specialized nuclear cardiology departments, or in general nuclear medicine departments with a high throughput of cardiac cases.

Gated SPECT and attenuation correction

Gating is available on any contemporary SPECT camera. Attenuation correction is available on many gamma cameras, whether using a scanning gadolinium source(s) or X-ray computed tomography (CT). The latter tends to be more expensive to purchase, though the former requires regular replacement of the source(s).

Specific quality control issues

- Gantry.
- Centre of rotation.
- Uniformity.
- Stability of uniformity at different angles.
- Total performance (Jaszczak) phantom.

Acquisition options

Orbit

- 180° (right anterior oblique to left posterior oblique) versus 360°.
- Contoured versus circular.
- Number of angular projections (32 versus 64).

Size of image matrix

- Usually 64 × 64.

SPECT reconstruction: filtered back-projection

Filtered back-projection is the commonest method used to reconstruct a SPECT acquisition.

Back-projection (see Fig. 4.1)

Individual transaxial slices are reconstructed from corresponding rows of pixels on each planar projection. The count value of each pixel in a row corresponds to the total activity along a line perpendicular to the camera face. A constant value is assumed for each point along the line, and is back-projected onto a digital image matrix. This is repeated for each pixel in the row for each projection.

The result is a blurred image of a transaxial slice: regions of higher activity are seen against a noisy background, with prominent 'star artefacts'. Filtering is therefore required to improve image quality by enhancing the signal and suppressing the noise.

Filtering

Filters are best considered in the frequency domain rather than in the more familiar spatial domain. Fourier analysis is used to describe the image in terms of its spatial frequencies, in units of cycles per pixel. In these terms, low frequency data contain most of the structural information. High frequency data provide detail in the image (edges etc.), but also represent noise. The challenge of filtering is therefore to remove high frequency noise without losing detail. Filters are described by the frequencies that they transmit:

- Low-pass filters transmit only low frequencies and smooth an image at the expense of detail.
- High-pass filters accentuate detail but produce a grainy image.

Filtered back-projection requires two filters (see Fig. 4.2):
- Ramp filter.
- Smoothing filter.

The ramp filter is used to correct the smoothing effect of the back-projection process itself, and remove star artefact. Each spatial frequency is amplified in proportion to its magnitude up to a maximum frequency. A smoothing filter (often a Butterworth or Hanning filter) is then required to remove the high frequency noise enhanced by the ramp filter. This can be described in terms of its:

- Cut-off, the frequency at which the magnitude falls to 50%: this must be sufficiently high to include all true image data, or an over-smoothed image will be produced.
- Roll-off, represented by the order, the slope at 50% magnitude: this suppresses artefacts.

The choice of smoothing filter varies from department to department, and is usually made empirically to provide the best images from a given camera and processing software, with a given type and dose of radiopharmaceutical. Once chosen, the same filter should be used for all patient studies.

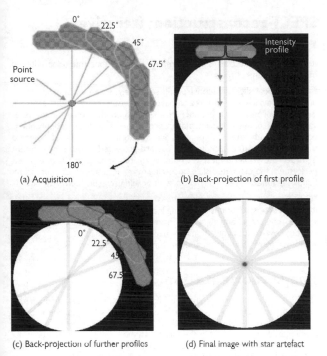

(a) Acquisition

(b) Back-projection of first profile

(c) Back-projection of further profiles

(d) Final image with star artefact

Fig. 4.1 Back-projection following SPECT acquisition of a point source (see text).

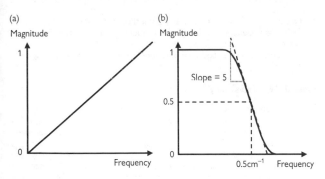

Fig. 4.2 Filters used in filtered back-projection. (a) Ramp filter; (b) Butterworth filter with cut-off 0.5cm^{-1} and order 5.

SPECT reconstruction: iterative reconstruction

Iterative reconstruction is an alternative to the more traditional filtered back-projection.

Each transaxial slice is reconstructed separately. As an initial estimate, all pixels in the slice are assumed to have equal count density. This estimate is forward-projected to produce an expected count profile for the relevant line of pixels on each planar projection. This expected profile is compared with the real profile, and the transverse slice is adjusted slightly. The updated slice is again forward-projected, another adjustment is made, and so on until a set number of iterations (e.g. 30) have been performed, the estimated slice becoming more accurate on each occasion. Following iterative reconstruction, a smoothing (e.g. Butterworth) filter is applied.

Iterative reconstruction is becoming increasingly popular:
• Faster computers and algorithms have made it practical for everyday use.
• Noisy low-count acquisitions are handled more reliably.
• Non-uniform attenuation and photon scatter can be corrected.

Image reorientation

SPECT reconstruction produces a set of transverse slices through the heart perpendicular to the long axis of the body, which can be used to generate sets of sagittal and coronal slices. The long axis of the left ventricle is orientated obliquely within the thorax, so the images are reorientated to produce slices which pass perpendicularly through the major myocardial walls (see Fig. 4.3). Most modern processing software does this automatically:
• Vertical long axis: the central transverse slice is identified, and a set of slices is produced parallel to and including the long axis of the left ventricle.
• Horizontal long axis: the central sagittal slice is identified, and a set of slices is produced parallel to and including the long axis of the left ventricle.
• Short axis: slices are produced perpendicular to the horizontal long axis.

Colour display

The count density of each pixel within the reorientated slices is displayed relative to the pixel of maximal counts in the myocardium (0–100%) using a greyscale or colour spectrum. Many colour scales are available commercially, but continuous scales are preferable (e.g. 'GE cool', as used in this book) as they avoid abrupt changes in colour between regions with only small differences in count density. Occasionally, automated processing results in incorrect normalization to extracardiac activity abutting the heart, so that the entire myocardium appears artefactually 'cold'. In such cases, manual correction is required.

SPECT studies should be reported from a computer workstation, not from a hard copy. A number of formats are available for displaying the processed slices. Conventionally, all slices are displayed simultaneously as follows:
- Top panel: short axis slices with stress above rest, from apex on left to base on right.
- Middle panel: vertical long axis slices with stress above rest, from septum on left to lateral wall on right.
- Bottom panel: horizontal long axis slices with stress above rest, from inferior wall on left to anterior wall on right.

Some readers prefer to view a more limited number of slices at a time, scrolling between slices in a given plane. This may be combined with quantitative images on the same display, depending on the software.

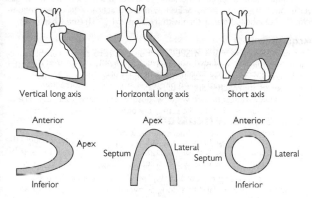

Fig. 4.3 Standard orthogonal planes used in SPECT.

Gated SPECT: acquisition and reconstruction

SPECT acquisitions can be gated to the electrocardiogram in a similar way to equilibrium radionuclide ventriculography (see Chapter 5). The planar projections are acquired as 8 or 16 frames, and each frame is reconstructed separately to produce slices which represent the left ventricle at a particular point in the cardiac cycle. Static slices to assess perfusion can be obtained from the same acquisition by summing the frames for each planar projection.

Each gated frame contains only one-eighth or one-sixteenth of the counts in an equivalent ungated acquisition, and so when used in myocardial perfusion scintigraphy gated SPECT is more practical with a technetium-99m (^{99m}Tc)-labelled tracer than with thallium-201 (^{201}Tl) (see Chapter 8).

Acquisition

The main challenge in gated SPECT acquisition is to obtain reliable functional information without rejecting excessive numbers of beats that would compromise the quality of the more important perfusion data. A number of approaches are used:

- Set a wide R-R acceptance window: ensures that almost all beats are acquired, but functional indices may become unreliable if significant R-R variation.
- Set a narrow (e.g. 20%) R-R acceptance window: ensures reliable functional information, but perfusion data compromised if excessive beat rejection; to address this
  - Each projection can be acquired for a set period of 'live' time (i.e. not including rejected beats), which can accommodate a degree of R-R variability as long as overall acquisition time not impractically long.
  - An extra 'frame' can be created for the rejected beats, which can be added into the summed data used to reconstruct the static perfusion slices.

Most commonly, 8 frames per cardiac cycle are used, though some departments prefer 16. Reducing the number of frames increases counts and hence quality of each frame, but reduces temporal resolution. As a result, ejection fraction calculated from an 8-frame study is typically a little lower than that from a 16-frame study due to overestimation of end-systolic volume.

Reconstruction and processing

A gated SPECT acquisition is reconstructed frame by frame and reorientated in a similar way to an ungated acquisition. Slices can be viewed in a looped cine format to assess regional function in terms of wall excursion and thickening. As a result of the limited spatial resolution of SPECT and the partial volume effect, the latter is seen as increasing count density.

Commercially available software can be used to fit endocardial and epicardial boundaries using a combination of count profile across the myocardial walls and geometric modelling. The left ventricular cavity volume is determined for each frame, and end-diastolic volume, end-systolic volume and ejection fraction are derived.

Attenuation correction

Soft tissue attenuation is a challenge to reliable reporting in SPECT. The experienced reader learns to 'read around' most such artefacts using the raw data and gated SPECT as aids, but in certain cases it is impossible to distinguish between a real defect and attenuation artefact. In order to reduce uncertainty, attenuation correction (AC) is increasingly available.

A *transmission* acquisition is performed using one or more scanning gadolinium sources or X-ray CT, and an attenuation map is reconstructed. This is used to correct the *emission* acquisition which is acquired simultaneously (gadolinium approach) or separately (CT approach). Different manufacturers employ a wide range of strategies, and a reader must be satisfied as to validity of the AC used in his/her own department.

Procedure

Transmission imaging involves positioning a source of radiation on one side of the patient and detecting the transmitted photons on the other. The ideal transmission source would emit photons of an energy which is:
- Uniform.
- Lower than the photon energy of the emission source (^{99m}Tc or ^{201}Tl) to avoid contaminating the SPECT acquisition.
- Sufficiently close to the photon energy of the emission source so that the attenuation map is applicable without excessive correction.

Gadolinium-153 (^{153}Gd) emits photons at 97 and 103keV, and is used in sealed transmission sources to correct ^{99m}Tc SPECT in a number of commercially available systems:
- Scanning line source with parallel-hole collimator.
- Multiple line sources with parallel-hole collimator.
- Scanning point source with any low-energy collimator.

More recently, X-ray CT has been introduced commercially for AC. CT provides excellent count statistics and a high quality attenuation map, but is performed separately from the SPECT acquisition. This gives the potential for misregistration between the transmission and emission data.

Challenges of using AC

AC should only be used in experienced departments with experienced readers, as it poses challenges of its own in terms of
- Expense.
- Gamma camera servicing and quality control.
- Image acquisition, particularly accurate registration between emission and transmission scans.
- Processing and reporting, with extra steps involved and a new range of normal appearances to be learned.

Ensuring high quality SPECT

SPECT acquisition requires a patient to lie supine with the left arm above the head for at least 15 minutes. Patient movement is a common but potentially avoidable cause of suboptimal image quality. Repetition of acquisitions is uncomfortable for the patient and inconvenient for the smooth running of a department. Moreover, repeat imaging is not an option following a poor quality stress ^{201}Tl acquisition. Clear instructions to the patient and attention to detail when setting up the acquisition significantly reduces the chance of poor quality images.

Setting up acquisition

- Time the scan appropriately, depending on tracer and method of stress used, to reduce problems with liver/gut activity.
- For women, ensure brassiere on or off, with or without strapping, according to departmental protocol; strapping may reduce anterior attenuation, but it is probably more important that the breasts be in the same position for stress and rest imaging.
- Ensure no metal objects (e.g. coins, keys, nitrate spray) in top pocket.
- Ensure head configuration, collimators, acquisition parameters *etc.* appropriate to radionuclide, dose, and type of study.
- Scrutinize electrocardiographic monitor if SPECT to be gated, to ensure sufficient regularity.
- Position heads so that they remain as close as possible to patient throughout orbit, but without danger of collision.
- Position heart within field of view on each projection, especially apex.
- Following acquisition, scrutinize raw data and preferably reconstruct the acquisition before the patient leaves the department: it is much easier to repeat a poor quality acquisition at this stage than to bring the patient back for a complete repeat study.

Patient comfort

- Explain what will happen, and requirement to relax, lie still, and not talk.
- Provide environment in which patient can remain relaxed but awake, with steady heart rate: for example, no background conversation, relaxing music.
- Maximize comfort in supine position: for example, provide hand grips above head, support under head, support under knees to relax lower back.
- Light strapping to remind the patient to lie still may be helpful.

Radionuclide ventriculography

Introduction

Radionuclide ventriculography (RNV) was the first reliable non-invasive method of assessing left ventricular (LV) function, and established nuclear cardiology as a clinical discipline. The subsequent development of other imaging modalities, particularly echocardiography, has led to a sharp decline in the number of studies performed, but RNV still has a role in situations where reproducible serial assessments of LV ejection fraction are required.

RNV is performed using a *first-pass* or, much more commonly, an *equilibrium* method. The first-pass method (FPRNV) involves following a bolus of injected radiopharmaceutical on its first transit through the heart. It can provide accurate information about both RV and LV function, as well as intracardiac shunts, but is technically very demanding. Equilibrium RNV (ERNV) is straightforward and much more commonly performed. It involves radionuclide labelling of the blood pool (i.e. with the radiopharmaceutical dose at 'equilibrium'), followed by summation of several hundred cardiac cycles. ERNV provides an accurate measurement of LV ejection fraction only.

A word on terminology

A confusing array of alternative names for the investigation here termed RNV appear in the literature. The popular term 'MUGA' (multi-gated acquisition) scan should no longer be used as it refers to an outdated method of acquiring equilibrium RNV images.

Most of the alternative names comprise three elements:
- 'First-pass', or 'equilibrium' and/or 'blood-pool', referring to the method being used.
- 'Radionuclide', as distinct from invasive contrast ventriculography.
- 'Ventriculography', or 'angiography', or 'angiocardiography', or 'cineangiography', or even 'cineangiocardiography' (!), referring to the image acquisition and display.

In an attempt to impose consistency, the American College of Cardiology and American Heart Association have chosen the names first-pass radionuclide angiography (FPRNA) and equilibrium radionuclide angiography (ERNA). However, the term RNV represents a more accurate description of the investigation, and is preferred here.

ERNV: blood-pool labelling

ERNV is performed after labelling the blood pool with ^{99m}Tc. Originally, labelled human serum albumin (HSA) was used, but direct labelling of the red blood cells with ^{99m}Tc-pertechnetate has largely superceded this.

^{99m}Tc-pertechnetate diffuses passively into red cells and, in the presence of preadministered stannous ions (Sn^{2+}), is reduced and binds with haemoglobin β-chains. Three labelling techniques may be employed:

In vivo technique

- Inject stannous pyrophosphate 10–20µg per kg body weight intravenously.
- 10–30 minutes later, inject ^{99m}Tc-pertechnetate 800MBq (UK dose; confers 7mSv).

This is the simplest and most widely practised method. Its disadvantage is a relatively low labelling efficiency (85–95%), though this is entirely adequate for clinical purposes.

In vitro technique

- Take blood sample and incubate with stannous.
- Separate red cells by centrifugation and reincubate with ^{99m}Tc-pertechnetate.
- Wash labelled cells and resuspend.
- Reinject into patient.

This technique provides optimal labelling efficiency (100%), but involves handling of blood and is complex and time-consuming.

Modified *in vivo* technique

- Inject stannous pyrophosphate 10–20µg per kg body weight intravenously.
- 10–30 minutes later, draw an aliquot of blood into a syringe containing an anticoagulant and the dose of ^{99m}Tc-pertechnetate.
- Incubate at room temperature for 10–20 minutes with occasional agitation.
- Reinject into patient.

This technique offers a compromise between the simplicity of the *in vivo* approach and the labelling efficiency of the *in vitro* approach (90–95% for modified *in vivo*).

ERNV: principles of ECG-gating

Given the relatively low radioactivity that can be conferred on the blood pool, acquiring an image with an acceptable number of counts requires several minutes, and cardiac function cannot be visualized cycle-by-cycle in real time. It is therefore necessary to 'gate' image acquisition to a patient's electrocardiogram (ECG) in order to preserve timing information in the final acquisition.

Types of gating

Frame mode

This is the commonest approach. Each R-R interval on the ECG is divided into a fixed number of frames (16–32, depending on the purpose of the study). Counts from equivalent frames of several hundred successive cardiac cycles are summed in the same image (see Fig. 5.1). The result is a set of images, each representing a particular phase of the cardiac cycle, which can be played as a cine loop and processed as required.

List mode

This is less commonly performed, as historically it was difficult to handle the large amount of data with the computer memory available. The acquisition is stored as a list of the X and Y coordinates of every detected scintillation, together with timing data from the ECG. This method allows great flexibility in subsequent processing, though in practice this is unnecessary for most routine indications.

Beat rejection

Gating assumes that all cardiac cycles are of equal length, and hence have equivalent diastolic filling time and ejection fraction. It is therefore desirable to exclude from the acquisition R-R intervals which deviate markedly from the average, commonly the interval on either side of an extrasystole. This can be done by setting an R-R acceptance window (typically the mean ±10%). This makes ERNV unsuitable for patients with irregular atrial fibrillation or very frequent extrasystoles.

ERNV: acquisition

- ECG electrodes are applied and connected to the camera to allow gating.
- For quantification of global LV function, planar 45° left anterior oblique (LAO) acquisition allows LV to be viewed relatively free of overlap from right ventricle or atria; angle may need to be varied to ensure adequate septal separation between ventricles; 20° of caudal tilt (if camera allows) may avoid atrial overlap.
- Using frame mode (16 frames adequate for ejection fraction), acquisition continues until 100 000–200 000 counts per frame achieved.
- For full assessment of regional LV function, additional projections are necessary, typically anterior or 30° right anterior oblique view, and left lateral view.

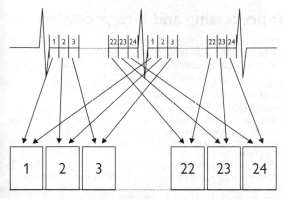

Fig. 5.1 Principle of frame-mode gating.

ERNV: processing and interpretation (1)

Cine loops

Cine loops of the available projections are inspected. With experience, a good visual assessment of both global and regional LV function can be made.

Left ventricular ejection fraction

Left ventricular ejection fraction is calculated from the LAO view (see Fig. 5.2). The same validated automated computer software should be used whenever possible to ensure reproducibility. Manual drawing of regions of interest should be reserved for cases where the computer algorithm has failed.

- Region of interest (ROI) is drawn around LV cavity on end-diastolic (maximal counts) and end-systolic (minimal counts) frames, and counts measured within each.
- To correct for background counts from thoracic structures anterior and posterior to LV, crescent shaped background ROI is drawn just outside and inferolateral to end-diastolic LV ROI; care taken that this does not overlap spleen to avoid subsequent overcorrection; counts per pixel measured within background ROI.
- Assuming that measured counts are directly proportional to blood volume, dimensionless LV ejection fraction is given by formula

$$EF = \frac{\text{end-diastolic counts} - \text{end-systolic counts}}{\text{end-diastolic counts} - \text{background counts within LV ROI}}$$

In principle, this counts-based calculation of ejection fraction is independent of LV geometry and hence highly accurate. In practice, there are some important sources of error:

- Background activity hard to estimate accurately and reproducibly.
- Some degree of overlap with other cardiac chambers may be unavoidable.
- γ-photons arising from blood deeper (more inferiorly) within the LV cavity are more likely to be attenuated or scattered than those arising more superficially (anteriorly); thus anterior wall motion abnormality may have larger effect on calculated ejection fraction than equivalent inferior abnormality.

Absolute LV volumes can also be calculated using ERNV, but this involves a correction for attenuation and measurement of the count rate per ml of a blood sample and is seldom performed.

Right ventricular ejection fraction cannot be accurately assessed from planar ERNV because of overlap with the right atrium in the LAO projection, and with the LV in other projections.

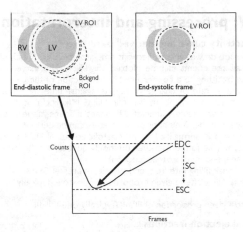

Fig. 5.2 Analysis of LAO ERNV acquisition (RV, right ventricle; LV, left ventricle; ROI, region of interest; EDC, end-diastolic counts within LV ROI; ESC, end-systolic counts within LV ROI; SC, stroke counts; bckgnd, background).

ERNV: processing and interpretation (2)

Time-activity curve and derived parameters

If LV ROIs are drawn on each frame, a time-activity curve (TAC) of frame number against counts can be plotted (Fig. 5.2). The curve is usually smoothed by fitting to a Fourier function. Inspection of the curve and its first derivative (rate of change of counts against time) provides useful information, particularly about diastolic filling. Meaningful assessment of diastolic function requires at least 32 frames if frame-mode is used, or preferably list-mode. A number of parameters can be derived:

- Peak filling rate, normalized as end-diastolic counts or stroke counts per second (the former is more commonly quoted, but the latter is more independent of systolic function).
- Time to peak filling rate from end-systole, expressed in ms.
- Fractional filling after a given proportion of diastole (typically one-third).
- Time to a given proportion of filling (typically one-third).

Regional ejection fractions

Regional LV function can be quantified by assigning a 'centre of gravity' to the LV ROI, and constructing a number of radial sectors of equal angle. The regional ejection fraction of each sector can then be calculated.

Parametric images

Regional function can also be studied on a pixel-by-pixel basis by generating static parametric images of *amplitude* and *phase*.

Each pixel has its own TAC, but the paucity of counts necessitates imperfect modelling to the first Fourier harmonic of time. This is a symmetrical cosine curve characterized by an amplitude (the depth of the fitted curve) and a phase angle (the timing in degrees of peak amplitude, i.e. end-diastole, within the cardiac cycle). Each pixel can be colour-coded for either amplitude or phase, and a pair of parametric images generated.

Phase images can be further analyzed by plotting a histogram of pixel phase angles for a ventricular ROI: the width of the distribution is a measure of contractile dyssynchrony, and can be expressed as a standard deviation (for a LV ROI, values below 12° are normal).

Parametric images have been valuable in assessing:
- Regional wall motion abnormalities in coronary disease, particularly LV aneurysms which unlike non-aneurysmal scar have amplitude (due to passive expansion in systole) but phase values similar to the atria (see Fig. 5.3).
- Conduction abnormalities, such as bundle branch blocks and pre-excitatory accessory pathways.
- Inter- and intraventricular dyssynchrony prior to biventricular pacing for heart failure.

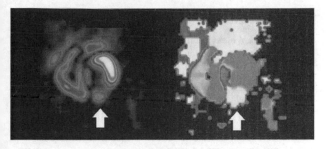

Fig. 5.3 Amplitude (left) and phase (right) images of left ventricular aneurysm (white arrow), which has amplitude but is 180° out of phase with the rest of the ventricle. (See colour plate section.)

Clinical value of ERNV

Accuracy of LV ejection fraction

Values of LV ejection fraction measured by ERNV are typically ≤5% lower than those measured by other modalities as a result of at least some atrial overlap. It is important for every department to define its own normal range and reproducibility for a given camera and processing algorithm. A typical lower limit of normal would be 50%.

The main strength of ERNV LV ejection fraction is its reproducibility, which should be ±5% between observers and between acquisitions. This makes it particularly suitable for clinical situations in which *changes* in ejection fraction over time are important.

Coronary disease and cardiomyopathies

Many landmark studies [e.g. the Coronary Artery Surgery Study (CASS) trial of bypass surgery] established ERNV ejection fraction as a key prognostic indicator in patients with coronary disease. In general, risk is low for LV ejection fraction above 40%, but increases exponentially as the value decreases below this threshold.

Echocardiography has largely replaced ERNV in the everyday assessment of LV function, except in the very occasional patient with impossible acoustic windows. Nevertheless, ERNV may still be of value in situations which call for an accurate ejection fraction to select patients for specific treatment options, for example, insertion of an implantable cardioverter-defibrillator (ICD).

Monitoring cardiac effects of chemotherapy

Cancer chemotherapy with anthracyclines such as doxorubicin can cause myocardial damage and LV dysfunction. The risk of damage is related to cumulative dose, and is only 2% below $300mg/m^2$, but rises to as much as 20% above $700mg/m^2$. Damage is irreversible, and progresses rapidly if treatment with doxorubicin is continued.

ERNV is a well validated method of monitoring chemotherapy patients for early evidence of LV dysfunction, and clear guidelines exist:
• Perform baseline ERNV.
• If baseline EF ≥50%:
  • 2nd ERNV 3 weeks after $250–300mg/m^2$
  • 3rd ERNV 3 weeks after $450mg/m^2$ (or $400mg/m^2$ if risk factors)
  • Sequential ERNV 3 weeks after each subsequent dose
  • If at any stage ejection fraction falls by ≥10% to level <50%, do not give any more doxorubicin.
• If baseline EF 30–50%:
  • Sequential ERNV 3 weeks after every dose
  • If at any stage ejection fraction falls by ≥10% or absolute value <30%, do not give any more doxorubicin.
• If baseline EF <30%:
  • Do not use doxorubicin.

SPECT ERNV

ERNV can be performed with SPECT rather than planar acquisition, using similar parameters to those used for gated perfusion SPECT. In principle, this avoids the problem of overlapping structures, and allows an accurate geometric calculation of both left and right ventricular ejection fraction using appropriate software.

Left ventricular ejection fraction using SPECT ERNV is typically 5% higher than using the planar technique.

In practice, the advantages of SPECT ERNV have been insufficient to displace the simpler planar approach.

Exercise ERNV

The reproducibility of RNV makes it particularly suitable for the assessment of global LV function during exercise. In the past, both exercise FPRNV and exercise ERNV were widely used for the investigation of patients with known or suspected coronary disease. However, the development of myocardial perfusion scintigraphy (MPS) (particularly with gated SPECT) and stress echocardiography has led to a sharp decline in the number of exercise RNV studies performed.

ERNV is less technically demanding than FPRNV, particularly during exercise, and is more commonly performed. Strictly speaking, the prolonged acquisition times for the equilibrium method should lead to a less accurate measurement of peak exercise LV ejection fraction than the first-pass method, but in practice both techniques appear to yield equivalent clinical information.

Performing exercise ERNV

- Label the blood pool.
- Acquire resting anterior/RAO and left lateral projections, finishing with a LAO projection for LV ejection fraction.
- Monitor 12-lead ECG and blood pressure.
- Exercise is most conveniently performed with patient lying supine on camera table pedalling specially mounted bicycle ergometer; shoulder restraints and hand grips can help to stabilize upper body; upright ergometer exercise can also be used, but patient motion a bigger problem.
- Commence exercise at workload 25W, increasing by 25W every 3 minutes.
- Acquire LAO projections with wider R-R acceptance window than at rest (e.g. ±15% rather than ±10%), accepting fewer counts to shorten acquisition time (e.g. 120 000 rather than 150 000 counts per frame).
- Begin acquisitions at least 1 minute into each stage to allow stabilization of heart rate; obtain as many acquisitions as possible before patient reaches standard exercise test end-point; as peak exercise approaches, consider fixing or even reducing workload to keep patient exercising long enough to complete acquisition.

Treadmill exercise is almost impossible to combine with ERNV because of patient motion. Immediate post-treadmill imaging is unsatisfactory as LV ejection fraction tends to rebound back to or above the resting level on cessation of exercise, giving a misleadingly high value for exercise ejection fraction. In contrast to myocardial perfusion scintigraphy, pharmacological stress is an inadequate alternative to exercise when combined with ERNV as only patients with the most severe coronary disease demonstrate a fall in ejection fraction.

Value in known or suspected coronary disease

The response in a normal subject is a rise in LV ejection fraction of at least 5%.

In patients with coronary disease, the resting ejection fraction may be reduced if there is extensive infarction (and/or hibernating myocardium), whilst there may be a fall in ejection fraction if there is significant inducible ischaemia. The absolute ejection fraction during exercise encapsulates in a single index both types of information, and emerges as the most important single index in a number of studies.

In comparison to MPS with SPECT or stress echocardiography, single plane ERNV provides very limited regional wall motion information and may fail to demonstrate relatively minor (i.e. single vessel) coronary disease which is insufficient to affect global LV function. This is a problem in the straightforward diagnosis or exclusion of coronary disease, and so exercise ERNV is more suitable for assessing the overall extent of ischaemia and its consequent prognostic importance. A rise in ejection fraction or an exercise ejection fraction above 50% are reassuring. Conversely, a fall of 5% or more, or an absolute exercise ejection fraction of less than 30% are both associated with a high risk of cardiac death or nonfatal myocardial infarction. There is evidence that, in patients already known to have three vessel coronary disease, only those with a fall in ejection fraction of 8% or more derive prognostic benefit from bypass surgery.[1]

Value in asymptomatic aortic regurgitation

Exercise ERNV has also been used to assess contractile reserve in asymptomatic patients with significant aortic regurgitation. Such patients are usually managed conservatively until symptoms develop or echocardiographic evidence of LV systolic dysfunction appears (e.g. end-systolic dimension >55mm). In cases of uncertainty, exercise ERNV may provide additional useful information:

- Resting LV ejection fraction <45% is itself an indication for surgery.
- Fall in ejection fraction during exercise of >5% predicts high risk of death, onset of symptoms, or progression to resting dysfunction (13% per year), and may lower the threshold for surgery or prompt very close follow-up.[2]

References

1 Supino PG, Borer JS, Herrold FM, et al. Prognostication in 3-vessel coronary artery disease based on left ventricular ejection fraction during exercise: influence of coronary artery bypass grafting. Circulation 1999; 100: 974–32.

2 Borer JS, Hochreiter C, Herrold EM, et al. Prediction of indications for valve replacement among asymptomatic or minimally symptomatic patients with chronic aortic regurgitation and normal left ventricular performance. Circulation 1998; 97: 525–34.

First-pass radionuclide ventriculography

Performing FPRNV

FPRNV can be performed following injection of a bolus of any ^{99m}Tc-labelled radiopharmaceutical, most commonly ^{99m}Tc-pertechnetate during *in vivo* blood-pool labelling for ERNV, or a ^{99m}Tc-labelled perfusion tracer during MPS.

- Inject compact bolus of radiopharmaceutical (<1ml) through large cannula in right antecubital vein, followed by 10–20ml saline flush.
- Image with appropriate gamma camera able to cope with high count rates (>150 000 counts per second), fitted with high sensitivity collimator.
- Acquire in list mode, or more commonly in an ECG-gated dynamic mode:
  - Right ventricular function: 30° RAO projection, 2000 × 25ms frames
  - Left ventricular function: anterior projection, 2000 × 25ms frames
  - Shunt quantification: anterior projection, 2000 × 50ms frames
- Check bolus adequate by measuring counts within ROI over superior vena cava: full width at half maximum should be 2–3 seconds for right ventricular study, but <1 second for LV or shunt study.

Processing and interpreting FPRNV

In comparison to ERNV, processing of first-pass data is much less automated and requires a significant amount of operator intervention for reliable results.

Right and left ventricular function

FPRNV remains the best radionuclide technique for assessing right ventricular ejection fraction, but is inferior to the equilibrium technique for LV function (count rates are substantially lower, and only one projection is available for assessment of regional function).

- Draw appropriate ventricular ROI, and construct TAC: shows peaks and troughs representing end-diastole and end-systole respectively as bolus traverses right ventricle, or arrives in LV having passed through the lungs.
- Select a few representative cycles with end-diastolic counts >50% of the maximal end-diastolic count and sum in frame mode for ejection fraction; use background correction for LV ejection fraction.

Quantification of left-to-right shunts

The role of FPRNA in the quantification of left-to-right shunts has been substantially reduced by modern echocardiography.

- Draw ROI over a lung field (right for intracardiac shunt, left for patent ductus arteriosus), and construct TAC: prior to recirculation there is normally a sharp rise and fall in count-rate, which are monoexponential; with left-to-right shunt, pulmonary washout is prolonged.

- Fit exponential curve to washout phase on raw data; subtract area under this primary fitted curve from raw data to leave area representing shunt component, and fit to secondary shunt curve.
- Calculate $Q_p:Q_s$ from

$$\frac{\Sigma \text{ area under primary and secondary curves}}{\text{area under primary curve}}$$

Introduction to myocardial perfusion scintigraphy

Introduction

Myocardial perfusion scintigraphy (MPS) is used to image relative myocardial blood flow at rest and during stress, thereby defining flow-limiting epicardial coronary stenoses and sometimes microvascular disease. It is commonly used diagnostically in patients with suspected coronary disease, and provides valuable prognostic information even in patients with proven disease.

A radiopharmaceutical perfusion tracer is injected during cardiac stress, and is taken up and retained by cardiac myocytes in relation to blood flow. Subsequent imaging is performed on a gamma camera, usually with single photon emission computed tomography (SPECT), and the distribution of radionuclide reflects myocardial viability and perfusion at the time of tracer injection, that is, during stress. A second imaging study is performed after injection of tracer at rest (^{99m}Tc-labelled tracers) or following redistribution of the stress injection (^{201}Tl), and the distribution of radionuclide primarily reflects viability. An area of reduced stress uptake but normal resting uptake (reversible perfusion defect) usually indicates viable myocardium supplied through a flow-limiting coronary stenosis. An area of reduced stress *and* rest uptake (fixed perfusion defect) usually indicates scar following myocardial infarction.

A word on terminology

The investigation termed MPS in this book has a plethora of alternative names, reflecting the large number of possible combinations of radiopharmaceutical, stress method and imaging technique (planar or SPECT). Thus, depending on the hospital, a patient might be referred for an 'exercise thallium scan', an 'adenosine tetrofosmin/Myoview scan', a 'dipyridamole/ Persantin sestamibi (mibi) scan', a 'planar thallium scan', a 'mibi SPECT scan', etc. In practice, the choice of tracer and stress method will be made by the Nuclear Medicine Department, often on the day of the test, and such names are unhelpful and misleading.

The term 'myocardial perfusion *imaging*' is frequently used, but a more specific name is required now that perfusion imaging can be performed using myocardial contrast echocardiography and cardiac magnetic resonance imaging. Thus we prefer the phrase 'myocardial perfusion *scintigraphy*', which reflects the particular form of imaging used in nuclear cardiology.

Stress testing for myocardial perfusion scintigraphy

Coronary physiology and stress testing

Normal coronary anatomy and physiology

The coronary arterial system consists of two functional parts:

- Epicardial coronary arteries: range in diameter from several millimetres down to about 400µm; do not normally exert significant resistance to blood flow.
- Microvasculature: arterioles and capillaries; modulate blood flow by varying their resistance over a five-fold range.

In contrast to most tissues, myocardial oxygen extraction is high (approximately 60%) at rest, and cannot increase significantly when demand increases during exercise. The necessary increase in myocardial oxygen uptake can only be achieved by a virtually linear increase in myocardial perfusion (see Fig. 7.1).

Coronary physiology in the presence of epicardial stenoses

In the presence of a significant epicardial coronary stenosis, the arterioles distal to the lesion vasodilate to compensate for the resistance it offers. Myocardial perfusion at rest remains normal until an epicardial stenosis is severe (80–85% by diameter, 60–80% by area). The myocardial uptake of a radiopharmaceutical perfusion tracer injected at rest is therefore homogeneous in the absence of myocardial infarction or critical coronary stenoses.

The use of vasodilator reserve to maintain resting perfusion limits the maximal coronary flow which can be achieved during exercise, to a degree which depends on the severity of the stenosis. Thus stress perfusion becomes heterogeneous in the presence of significant coronary disease, with myocardium subtended by stenosed arteries achieving lower levels than myocardium subtended by unobstructed arteries. The myocardial uptake of a radiopharmaceutical perfusion tracer injected during stress reflects this heterogeneity, with regions of relatively lower myocardial perfusion and tracer uptake appearing as 'inducible' or 'reversible' defects on imaging that are not present at rest.

Effect of different stress methods on flow

Stress using direct coronary vasodilators such as dipyridamole and adenosine provokes a four- to five-fold increase in flow within a normal coronary territory. Stress using exercise and dobutamine provokes coronary vasodilatation as a secondary effect of increased myocardial oxygen demand, and smaller increases in flow are achieved (two- to three-fold). In principle, the vasodilators should produce the greatest heterogeneity in perfusion between normal and abnormal coronary territories, and ought to be the optimal form of stress. In practice the plateauing of the relationship between perfusion and uptake for the available tracers erodes this advantage, so that the different methods of stress produce equivalent perfusion defects.

Inducible hypoperfusion versus ischaemia

Ischaemia is a metabolic phenomenon which occurs when myocardial oxygen demand exceeds coronary supply. During stress testing with exercise or dobutamine it occurs when myocardial perfusion distal to a coronary stenosis is unable to increase sufficiently to meet the increasing oxygen demand. The detection of ischaemia in terms of chest pain, ST changes on the electrocardiogram, or new wall motion abnormalities forms the basis of the exercise electrocardiogram or stress echocardiography, but is not the primary aim of myocardial perfusion scintigraphy. Indeed primary vasodilator stress seldom produces ischaemia, as heterogeneous perfusion occurs in the absence of increased myocardial oxygen demand. Nevertheless, vasodilator stress does occasionally provoke true ischaemia by a steal effect, via collaterals from a low-flow abnormal capillary bed into a high-flow normal coronary territory.

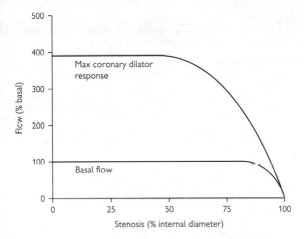

Fig. 7.1 Relation between coronary stenosis severity and flow at rest and during maximal coronary vasodilatation.

Practical requirements for stress testing

Stress room

In order to deliver myocardial perfusion scintigraphy as a high volume service it is important that patients be stressed efficiently as well as safely. Ideally the nuclear medicine/nuclear cardiology department should have its own in-house stress room, equipment and staff to minimize delays caused by 'borrowing' any of these from the cardiology department. The stress room should be:

- Easily accessible in case of emergency.
- Located close to camera room to facilitate rapid imaging when ^{201}Tl used.
- Large enough to accommodate necessary equipment.
- Air-conditioned.

A second room to prepare patients prior to stress, or allow prolonged recovery afterwards is an advantage if space permits.

Stress equipment

- Couch: for clinical assessment, pharmacological stress, and recovery after exercise.
- 12-lead electrocardiogram (ECG) machine: ideally with a system that can be pre-programmed for different stress protocols, with automatic printing at different stages.
- Manual sphygmomanometer and/or automated blood pressure machine: the latter can be prone to inaccuracy during exercise, but is convenient for pharmacological stress.
- Treadmill and/or bicycle ergometer.
- Rapid infusion syringe pump: for pharmacological stress; ideally should have facility to calculate infusion rates automatically from drug concentration and patient weight.
- Storage unit(s) for
  - Stress drugs and their antagonists
  - ECG electrodes
  - Consumables needed for venous cannulation, syringes, etc.
- Resuscitation trolley: with defibrillator and emergency drugs and equipment.

Stress personnel

Stress should be supervised by at least two members of staff. At least one of these should have a sound knowledge of the principles and practice of cardiac stress testing, and be trained and currently certified in cardiopulmonary resuscitation (in the UK, to Intermediate or preferably Advanced Life Support level; see Fig. 7.2). Where the main supervisor is a nurse or technologist, a physician should be immediately available to attend in problematic cases. The two members of staff should have clearly defined roles during the stress test in terms of patient monitoring, radiopharmaceutical injection, etc.

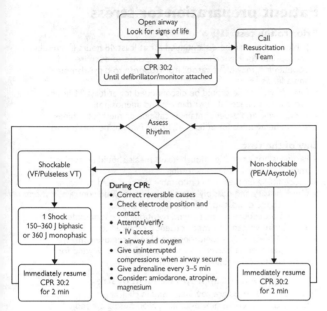

Fig. 7.2 Current Advanced Life Support (ALS) protocol.

Patient preparation for stress

Prior to the test

- β-blockers should be discontinued for at least 48 hours if clinically appropriate (prevent chronotropic response to exercise and dobutamine, may blunt vasodilator response to dipyridamole and adenosine).
- Oral dipyridamole should be discontinued for at least 24 hours (potentiates effects of dipyridamole and adenosine).
- Food, drink, and drugs containing caffeine or methylxanthines should be avoided for at least 12 hours (adenosine antagonists).

Day of the test

- Fasting is not desirable, though heavy meals should be avoided immediately prior to stress testing.
- Loose-fitting clothes and comfortable shoes should be worn.
- Quick history and possibly examination to exclude contraindications and determine most appropriate form of stress.
- Explain procedure to the patient, mentioning possible side effects, and obtain written informed consent if required locally.
- Set up 12-lead ECG monitoring and blood pressure cuff.
- Insert peripheral intravenous cannula, with three-way tap for pharmacological stress.

Choosing the most appropriate form of stress

Three forms of stress are routinely used in clinical practice:
- Exercise: most commonly dynamic/isotonic using a treadmill or bicycle ergometer.
- Vasodilator drug: dipyridamole or adenosine.
- Inotropic drug: currently only dobutamine.

In choosing the most appropriate form of stress for a given patient, the referral letter should be carefully scrutinized and a brief clinical assessment performed. All else being equal, exercise should be regarded as the first-line method of stress unless:
- Contraindicated.
- ECG shows left bundle branch block or ventricular pacing.
- Obvious that patient will be unable to achieve target heart rate.

For such patients, and those in whom exercise stress has been attempted unsuccessfully, a vasodilator drug (dipyridamole or adenosine) is the second choice. If a vasodilator is contraindicated (most commonly due to airways disease), dobutamine should be used.

It should be noted that, in order to streamline patient throughput, some centres have adopted dipyridamole or adenosine stress as their first-line method.

Exercise stress: general considerations

Introduction

Exercise is the most physiological form of cardiac stress and there is a vast literature confirming its effectiveness in the setting of myocardial perfusion scintigraphy. Exercise indices emerge as additional predictors of prognosis in most studies. Compared with pharmacological methods, image quality following exercise is usually superior due to splanchnic vasoconstriction and skeletal muscle vasodilatation which ensures that a smaller proportion of the injected dose appears in the gut. Whilst pharmacological stress provides a good alternative in most patients, exercise is more logical for patients being investigated for inducible hypoperfusion in the absence of epicardial coronary disease, for example, anomalous coronary arteries, myocardial bridging, microvascular disease.

Physiology

Exercise may be dynamic (isotonic, e.g. treadmill or ergometer) or isometric (e.g. hand-grip test). During dynamic exercise testing, the heart rate, systolic blood pressure, and cardiac output increase progressively. The maximum achievable heart rate declines with increasing age; it is also lower in women than in men. Heart rate is the biggest determinant of myocardial oxygen demand, and so myocardial perfusion is virtually linearly related to heart rate: a doubling in heart rate leads to a three-fold increase in perfusion in the territory of an unobstructed epicardial coronary artery. Peak heart rate is generally higher using treadmill than ergometer exercise.

In patients with coronary disease, the haemodynamic changes during exercise are dependent on several factors, such as the extent of any ischaemia, left ventricular function and body position. Approximately 3% of patients with coronary disease, particularly those with left mainstem or three vessel disease, develop significant (≥20mmHg below rest) hypotension during exercise.

Value of exercise test indices

A full discussion of the interpretation and clinical significance of exercise testing is beyond the scope of this book. In the context of myocardial perfusion scintigraphy, exercise indices are not usually required to diagnose/exclude coronary disease, but are nevertheless valuable.

- The exercise test may aid reporting of the images, giving more or less significance to what would otherwise be equivocal findings, or providing a clue that significant ischaemia has been missed for technical reasons (see Fig. 7.3).
- The exercise test provides a symptomatic context to the images: a given reversible defect may have very different management implications in the setting of good exercise capacity and no limiting chest pain compared with limiting angina at low workload.
- Exercise testing provides independent prognostic information, though the specific index emerging from multivariate analysis varies between studies (see Fig. 7.4).

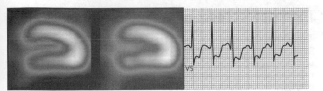

Fig. 7.3 Exercise test may aid reporting. This 62-year-old man underwent a one-day exercise-rest ^{99m}Tc-tetrosfosmin SPECT study. This demonstrated an equivocal reversible inferior perfusion defect which could easily have been dismissed as attenuation artefact (left panel shows representative vertical long axis slice, stress on left, rest on right). However the exercise test was strongly positive with limiting chest pain and deep ST depression at only 4 minutes of the Bruce protocol (right panel). Subsequent coronary angiography demonstrated a severe right coronary artery stenosis. (See colour plate section.)

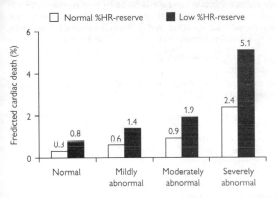

Fig. 7.4 Exercise indices provide independent prognostic information. The inability to achieve 80% of the predicted heart rate reserve

$$\frac{\text{peak heart rate} - \text{rest heart rate}}{(220 - \text{age}) - \text{rest heart rate}} \times 100$$

doubles cardiac mortality for any degree of abnormality of the SPECT images.[1]

References

1 Azarbal B, Hayes SW, Lewin HC, et al. The incremental prognostic value of percentage of heart rate reserve achieved over myocardial perfusion single-photon emission computed tomography in the prediction of cardiac death and all-cause mortality: superiority over 85% of maximal age-predicted heart rate. J Am Coll Cardiol 2004; **44**: 423–30.

Exercise stress: practical aspects

Treadmill exercise

Several treadmill exercise protocols are available, though the Bruce protocol is the most widely used in clinical practice (see Table 7.1). This is a multi-level exercise protocol and provides progressive increments in workload by increasing the speed and slope of the treadmill in a series of seven 3 minute stages. The modified Bruce protocol is a gentler version, with two additional stages at the beginning at the same speed as Bruce stage 1 but with smaller slopes. This slower increase in workload makes the modified Bruce protocol particularly suitable for older and frailer patients, and those who have previously performed poorly using the full Bruce.

Bicycle ergometer exercise

Bicycle ergometer exercise can be performed in upright, supine or semisupine positions. The exact protocol can be individualized to a patient's physical fitness and clinical state. A typical ergometer protocol involves the patient pedalling at a constant 50rpm against a progressively increasing load. Initial workload is usually 25W, increasing by 25W every 2–3 minutes.

Contraindications to exercise stress

Absolute contraindications

- Within 2–3 days of acute myocardial infarction.
- Uncontrolled unstable angina.
- Decompensated congestive heart failure.
- Uncontrolled hypertension (systolic blood pressure ≥200mmHg and/or diastolic blood pressure ≥115mmHg).
- Severe pulmonary hypertension.
- Endocarditis, myocarditis, or pericarditis.
- Acute aortic dissection.
- Acute pulmonary embolism or recent deep vein thrombosis.
- Uncontrolled cardiac dysrhythmias causing symptoms or haemodynamic compromise.

Relative contraindications

May be overridden if the value of exercise is believed to outweigh the risks.

- Significant left ventricular outflow tract obstruction (severe aortic stenosis or hypertrophic obstructive cardiomyopathy).
- Significant left mainstem stenosis.

Technical factors arguing against exercise

- Disabling non-cardiac medical problems likely to limit exercise capacity significantly.
- Left bundle branch block or ventricular pacing (associated with imaging artefacts).
- Failure to discontinue drugs likely to inhibit chronotropic response to exercise (β-blockers and/or certain calcium antagonists).

Table 7.1 Bruce and modified Bruce treadmill protocols

Stage	Time (minutes)	Speed (mph)	Slope (%)
0 (mod)	3	1.7	0
½ (mod)	3	1.7	5
1	3	1.7	10
2	3	2.5	12
3	3	3.4	14
4	3	4.2	16
5	3	5.0	18
6	3	5.5	20
7	3	6.0	22

Exercise stress: performing the test

Prior to the test

- β-blockers and, to a lesser extent, rate-limiting calcium antagonists should be discontinued for five half-lives (effectively 24–48 hours) prior to exercise testing; there is little evidence that this is harmful for stable patients.
- Fasting is not desirable, though heavy meals should be avoided immediately prior to exercise testing.
- Loose-fitting clothes and comfortable shoes should be worn.
- Quick history and possibly examination to exclude contraindications to exercise.
- Careful explanation and advice about exercise technique is essential to achieve optimal results, for example, for treadmill:
  - Long slow strides rather than short quick steps.
  - Rest hands on front bar, use it to stand up straight or even lean back.
  - Keep forward.
  - Give plenty of warning if starting to struggle to allow injection of tracer.
- Set up 12-lead ECG monitoring and blood pressure cuff, and insert peripheral intravenous cannula.
- Document heart rate, blood pressure, and record 12-lead ECG lying and standing prior to test.

During the test

- Commence exercise protocol: many treadmill and ergometer systems can be pre-programmed.
- Closely observe patient's state of comfort and ask about any chest pain.
- Continuously monitor ECG for ischaemic changes or dysrhythmias.
- Measure blood pressure 2 minutes into each stage.
- Record 12-lead ECG towards the end of each stage.
- Exercise testing should be patient/symptom-limited, unless there is a reason for early termination (see p. 87).
- Inject radiopharmaceutical followed by saline flush just prior to peak exercise, assuming:
  - Sustained achievement of target heart rate, that is, 85% of maximum predicted heart rate (220 − age for males, 210 − age for females), or
  - Limiting chest pain.
- Continue exercise for a further 1 minute following ^{201}Tl, or 2 minutes following ^{99m}Tc-labelled tracer.
- Record 12-lead ECG and measure blood pressure at peak exercise.
- Continue to monitor heart rate, blood pressure, and ECG for ≥4 minutes in recovery, or longer if chest pain or ischaemic ECG changes.

Report

- Protocol.
- Exercise time.
- Limiting symptom.

- Development of chest pain.
- Heart rate at rest and peak.
- Blood pressure at rest and peak.
- ECG at rest.
- ECG at peak exercise and into recovery.

Reasons for early termination of exercise test

- Patient needing to stop for any reason cardiac or non-cardiac: with experience a clinician learns to distinguish between the patient who *needs* to stop and the one who merely *asks* to stop but should be encouraged to continue.
- ST *elevation* of ≥1mm in leads without pathological Q-waves (excluding V1 and aVR): this suggests severe transmural ischaemia, and the leads involved indicate the ischaemic region on subsequent SPECT imaging (in contrast to ST depression).
- Progressive QRS broadening (as distinct from abrupt rate-dependent bundle branch block): this may indicate severe ischaemia.
- Significant dysrhythmia, or frequent ventricular ectopy in the setting of ischaemia.
- Fall in systolic blood pressure of ≥20mmHg below baseline with evidence of ischaemia.
- Excessive rise in blood pressure (systolic ≥250mmHg and/or diastolic ≥130mmHg).

NB: The development of ST depression of any severity need not be regarded as an absolute indication for early termination, though most protocols designed for technician-led stress have a 'bail-out' level (typically 3mm in the absence of angina, or 2mm in its presence).

Complications of exercise testing

Serious complications during exercise stress testing are uncommon. The risk is greatly influenced by the clinical situation, being higher in:
- Unstable angina.
- Left mainstem disease.
- Severe LV dysfunction.
- Critical aortic stenosis.
- History of serious dysrhythmia.

For the average patient, the following are reasonable approximations for the purposes of discussion:
- Death ≤1 in 10 000.
- Myocardial infarction or ventricular dysrhythmia 1 in 5000.

Vasodilator drugs: pharmacology

Introduction

Adenosine is a direct coronary vasodilator via its A_{2a} receptors, whilst dipyridamole acts indirectly by increasing the extracellular concentration of endogenous adenosine. Either provokes a four-fold increase in myocardial perfusion downstream of a normal epicardial coronary artery. Myocardial perfusion increases to a lesser degree downstream of a flow-limiting coronary stenosis. The result is heterogeneous perfusion between the territories of normal and stenosed coronary arteries, leading to a relative perfusion defect on myocardial perfusion scintigraphy. In most cases this occurs in the absence of metabolic ischaemia, as myocardial oxygen demand is not affected.

Physiology of adenosine

Adenosine is a ubiquitous substance that is produced in small amounts as part of normal cellular metabolism and in large amounts during tissue ischaemia and hypoxia. It is a small heterocyclic compound, composed of a purine base and the sugar ribose, with a molecular weight of 267Da (see Fig. 7.5).

Endogenous adenosine is produced intracellularly within vascular smooth muscle and endothelial cells via the ATP (adenosine triphosphate) and SAM (S-adenosyl methionine) pathways, or extracellularly by dephosphorylation of ATP and ADP (adenosine diphosphate) released from a variety of cell types. After extracellular release, adenosine re-enters cells through a facilitated transport mechanism where it is converted back into ATP and SAM, or is deaminated to inosine (which is eventually metabolized to urate).

Exogenously administered adenosine is rapidly taken up by cells, especially red blood cells and endothelial cells, which explains its remarkably short half-life.

Adenosine receptors

Extracellular adenosine interacts with a family of G-protein-coupled purine receptors located on cell membranes throughout the body (Fig. 7.6). Activation of A_2 receptors on vascular smooth muscle cells triggers production of adenylyl cyclase and cyclic AMP (adenosine monophosphate), which in turn results in the opening of potassium channels. This leads to hyperpolarization, with inhibition of intracellular calcium release and consequent smooth muscle relaxation. The result is arteriolar vasodilatation.

A_{2a} receptors are predominantly found in the coronary arterioles, and A_{2b} receptors in the systemic arterioles. A_{2b} receptors also mediate bronchoconstriction. Activation of A_1 receptors reduces the sinus rate and causes atrioventricular conduction delay, and triggers ischaemic preconditioning. A_3 and A_4 receptors are found on mast cells and may contribute to bronchospasm in susceptible persons.

Xanthines (methylxanthines and caffeine) are non-selective competitive antagonists of adenosine receptors.

Dipyridamole

Dipyridamole is a lipophilic pyrimidine base. It is excreted via the hepatobiliary route, and prolonged activity and side effects can be seen in hepatic insufficiency.

Dipyridamole inhibits the facilitated transport of adenosine into cells, raising the extracellular level of endogenous adenosine, which causes coronary vasodilatation. At high dosage dipyridamole is also a phosphodiesterase inhibitor, but it is unclear whether this contributes to its vasodilatory effect. It has antiplatelet actions, potentiating the effect of aspirin.

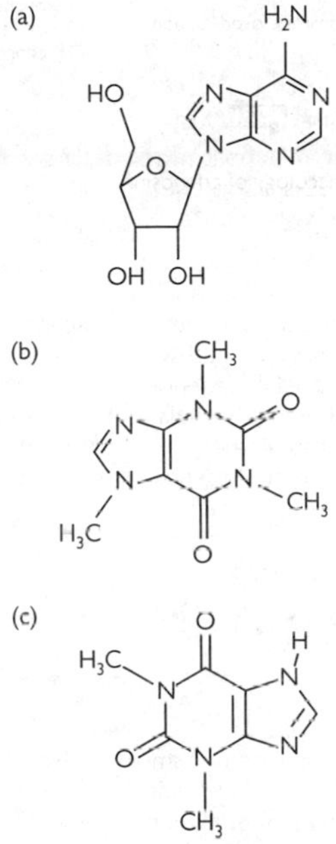

Fig. 7.5 Chemical structure of adenosine and its antagonists. (a) Adenosine; (b) caffeine; (c) theophylline.

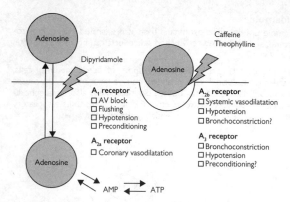

Fig. 7.6 Simplified pharmacology of adenosine.

Vasodilator drugs: practical considerations

Indications
- Inability to perform adequate exercise for physical or psychological reasons.
- Contraindication to exercise, for example, early (<5 days) after myocardial infarction.
- Left bundle branch block.
- Ventricular pacemaker.

Contraindications
- Confirmed acute coronary syndrome within 24 hours (once stabilized, vasodilator may be given depending on the clinical risk profile).
- Poorly controlled asthma with active wheeze (patients with unproven or well-controlled asthma may be given adenosine with caution, though dipyridamole should not be used because of the longer duration of side effects should they occur).
- Second- or third-degree atrioventricular block in the absence of a functioning pacemaker (patients with first-degree or intraventricular block can be given adenosine safely, though transient third-degree heart block is common in the former—1 in 7 compared with 1 in 100 normally).
- Significant sinoatrial disease in the absence of a functioning pacemaker.
- Baseline hypotension with systolic blood pressure <90mmHg.
- Xanthines (caffeine or methylxanthines) taken within 12 hours, or dipyridamole within 24 hours.

Caution should be exercised in patients with:
- Significant cerebrovascular disease, because hypotension may be hazardous.
- Heart transplant, who can be very sensitive to vasodilators due to cardiac denervation.

Haemodynamic effect of adenosine and dipyridamole
When infused intravenously, adenosine has an onset of action within a few seconds and a very short half-life of ≤10 seconds, primarily due to avid uptake by red blood cells. Coronary vasodilatation occurs within 1–2 minutes. At the usual dose of 140µg/kg/minute, maximal hyperaemia (typically a 4.4-fold increase in the resting level) is achieved in 92% of subjects. Even at a lower dose of 70µg/kg/minute it occurs in 84%.

The typical haemodynamic response to an adenosine infusion is a slight fall in systolic and diastolic blood pressure (mean 10mmHg), with a mild increase in heart rate (mean 10bpm) mediated by a reflex sympathetic response to peripheral vasodilatation.

Dipyridamole has similar effects to adenosine, but with a more delayed time-course. Maximal coronary vasodilatation does not occur until 3–4 minutes after intravenous injection, whilst its plasma half-life of 20–30 minutes makes its actions more prolonged.

Vasodilator drugs: performing the stress test

Prior to the test

- Oral dipyridamole should be discontinued for at least 24 hours.
- Food, drink, and drugs containing caffeine or methylxanthines should be avoided for at least 12 hours.
- Quick history and possibly examination to exclude contraindications.
- Weigh the patient.
- Explain procedure to the patient, mentioning likely side effects.
- Set up 12-lead ECG monitoring and blood pressure cuff.
- Insert peripheral intravenous cannula with three-way tap.

Standard 6-minute adenosine protocol

- Adenosine is available as 10ml vials of 3mg/ml solution (Adenoscan®); draw up 30ml (40ml for patients over 100kg) in a 50ml Luer-lock syringe, and attach via a giving-set to the three-way tap of the intravenous cannula.
- Record heart rate and blood pressure at baseline.
- Record a 12-lead ECG at baseline: look for resting atrioventricular and intraventricular conduction abnormalities.
- Give the adenosine infusion at a rate of 140µg/kg/minute over 6 minutes using a rapid infusion pump, together with exercise if possible (see below).
- Monitor the 12-lead ECG.
- Record heart rate, blood pressure, and a 12-lead ECG every 2 minutes during the infusion, or if a side effect develops.
- Three minutes into the infusion, inject the radiopharmaceutical via the three-way tap into the flowing stream of adenosine.
- Continue infusion for the final 3 minutes to flush in the radiopharmaceutical and maintain maximal coronary vasodilatation during myocardial uptake.
- Infusion should be discontinued early for any of the following:
  - Significant wheezing
  - Symptomatic, persistent high-grade atrioventricular block
  - Severe hypotension (systolic BP <80mmHg)
  - Severe chest pain associated with ≥2mm ST depression.

Adjustments to the standard adenosine protocol

Although often considered a contraindication, if a patient has had caffeine within the previous 12 hours adenosine can be given at an increased rate of 210µg/kg/minute to overcome the competitive antagonism.

If there is a history of unproven or well-controlled asthma, adenosine can be given cautiously at a reduced rate of 70µg/kg/minute for 30 seconds, increasing to 100µg/kg/minute for another 30 seconds and then to 140µg/kg/minute, if tolerated, for the final 5 minutes, with radiopharmaceutical injection at 4 minutes. The patient can be given two puffs of inhaled salbutamol prior to the infusion as an added precaution.

Abbreviated adenosine protocol

A 3–4 minute adenosine protocol, also at 140µg/kg/minute, combined with low-level exercise has also been used. The radiopharmaceutical is injected at 1.5–2 minutes.

Dipyridamole protocol

- Dipyridamole is available as 2ml vials containing 10mg of the drug (Persantin®); draw up the appropriate weight-related dose (0.56mg/kg) into a 10ml syringe; if required, the dose can be diluted with 0.9% saline or 5% dextrose in a larger syringe.
- Record heart rate and blood pressure at baseline.
- Record a 12-lead ECG at baseline: look for resting atrioventricular and intraventricular conduction abnormalities.
- Inject dipyridamole by hand over 4 minutes, followed by exercise if possible (see below).
- Monitor the 12-lead ECG.
- Record heart rate, blood pressure, and a 12-lead ECG every 2 minutes during the injection and for several minutes afterwards, or if a side effect develops.
- Three to four minutes *after* the dipyridamole injection, inject the radiopharmaceutical.

Combination with low-level exercise

Wherever possible (except early after an acute coronary syndrome, or in left bundle branch block or ventricular pacing), adenosine or dipyridamole stress should be combined with at least submaximal exercise. This reduces the incidence, intensity and duration of side effects, as well as improving image quality by reducing splanchnic uptake and increasing peripheral muscle uptake of radiopharmaceutical. Either ergometer or treadmill exercise can be used, and should be performed *during* an adenosine infusion, or *immediately after* a dipyridamole injection.

Vasodilator drugs: adverse effects

Adenosine

Minor adverse effects

Around 80% of patients have one or more adverse effects with adenosine. These are usually short-lived and mild, and rarely require specific treatment. The most common are:

- Flushing (40%).
- Chest pain (35%).
- Dyspnoea (35%).
- Headache (15%).
- Nausea (15%).
- Dizziness (10%).
- Symptomatic hypotension (5%).

Chest pain is caused by direct adenosine A_1-receptor stimulation independently of coronary disease. Dyspnoea is caused by stimulation of the carotid chemoreceptor with consequent hyperventilation.

Bronchoconstriction

With appropriate patient selection, serious bronchoconstriction is rare with adenosine (0.1%). It rarely requires reversal with aminophylline, a non-selective adenosine antagonist.

Atrioventricular block

First- and second-degree atrioventricular block are relatively common but are usually of minimal haemodynamic significance. Third-degree block occurs in approximately 1% of cases, though is commoner in those with first-degree block at baseline (15%), and requires either a decrease in rate or discontinuation of the infusion (see Fig. 7.7). Aminophylline is only rarely required (atropine is ineffective).

Ischaemia

Adenosine does not usually provoke ischaemia as it has little effect on myocardial oxygen demand. However, in some patients with severe coronary disease it may produce ischaemia via collateral-dependent and transmural steal effects. Therefore, significant ST segment depression is uncommon with adenosine (<10% of tests), but when present it is a strong predictor of severe coronary disease (sensitivity only 24%, but specificity 91%; see Fig. 7.8).

Death

Adenosine was not associated with any deaths in a series of nearly 10 000 cases. Anecdotal experience suggests that the mortality rate is probably of the same order as other forms of stress (1 in 10 000).

Dipyridamole

Dipyridamole causes similar adverse effects to adenosine, but somewhat less frequently (50%). They tend to occur following the injection, and may be prolonged (15–25 minutes). In contrast to adenosine, reversal with aminophylline is often required. Death has been reported only rarely with dipyridamole stress, and the risk appears no higher than with other forms of stress.

Reversal of vasodilator stress with aminophylline

Among its other pharmacological actions, aminophylline is a non-selective adenosine receptor antagonist. It is therefore useful in reversing adverse effects of dipyridamole or, much less commonly given the short half-life, adenosine. Aminophylline 75–100mg is given by *slow* intravenous injection, repeated if necessary.

Some departments administer aminophylline routinely to terminate dipyridamole stress 3–4 minutes after radiopharmaceutical injection.

NB: Aminophylline has no effect on the elevation of endogenous adenosine provoked by dipyridamole, so symptoms can sometimes recur after aminophylline has been metabolized.

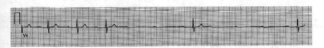

Fig. 7.7 Atrioventricular block during an adenosine infusion.

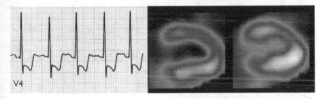

Fig. 7.8 Ischaemic ECG during an adenosine infusion (left panel). The patient was subsequently found to have a high-risk perfusion study (transient ischaemic dilatation and large reversible anteroapical perfusion defect, right panel), with severe multivessel coronary disease at angiography. (See colour plate section.)

Selective A$_{2a}$-receptor agonists

A number of selective adenosine A$_{2a}$ agonists have been developed for use in pharmacological stress: regadenoson, binodenoson, and apadenoson. These have the theoretical advantage of provoking maximal coronary vasodilatation without the A$_1$ and A$_{2b}$ mediated adverse effects seen with adenosine or dipyridamole. These compounds have longer half-lives than adenosine, and can therefore be administered as an intravenous bolus, further simplifying the stress test.

Regadenoson is currently the best evaluated agent in clinical trials:
- Diagnostic sensitivity equivalent to adenosine.
- Atrioventricular block and bronchoconstriction have not been reported.
- Minor adverse-effects still occur, though less frequently than with adenosine.
- Has been given safely to patients with airways disease.

Adenosine already has a good safety profile, even when used (with due caution) in patients with mild airways disease. It remains to be seen whether the additional advantages of selective adenosine A$_{2a}$ agonists such as regadenoson are sufficient to justify their widespread clinical use.

Dobutamine: pharmacology

Dobutamine is a synthetic catecholamine with positive inotropic and chronotropic effects on the heart (Fig. 7.9). It is a potent β_1-adrenoceptor agonist, with milder agonist activity at α_1- and β_2-receptors. The commercially available dobutamine preparation contains both the L-isomer, responsible for α_1 stimulation, and the D-isomer, responsible for β_1 and β_2 stimulation.

Low doses of dobutamine (up to 20µg/kg/minute) have a predominantly inotropic action via β_1 and α_1 activation. Higher doses induce a progressive chronotropic effect via α_1 activation. These inotropic and chronotropic effects increase myocardial oxygen demand, with secondary coronary vasodilatation. The increase in myocardial perfusion in the territory of an unobstructed coronary artery is comparable to that induced by exercise (two- to three-fold), but lower than with dipyridamole or adenosine.

In addition to its actions on the heart, dobutamine causes systemic vasodilatation via β_2 activation. Its effect on blood pressure is therefore variable between patients, depending on the balance between increasing cardiac output and falling systemic vascular resistance.

The onset of action of dobutamine occurs 1–2 minutes after starting an intravenous infusion, with the peak effect occurring about 10 minutes later. It has a short half-life (approximately 2 minutes) due to rapid metabolism (by catechol-o-methyltransferase) and conjugation in the liver.

(a)
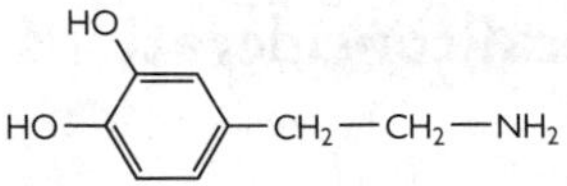

(b)
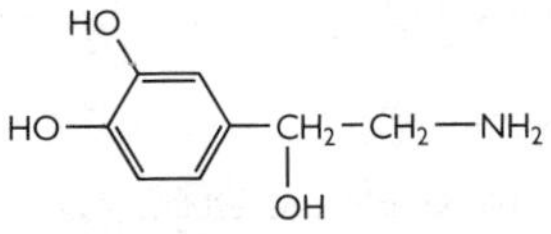

(c)
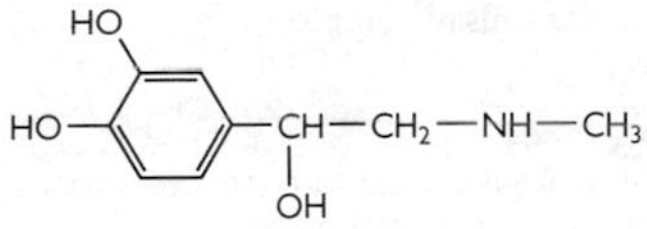

(d)
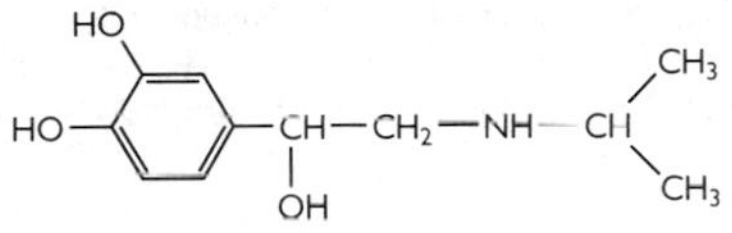

(e)
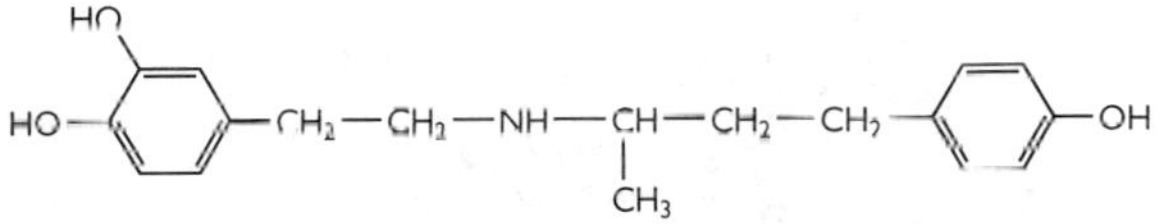

Fig. 7.9 Chemical structure of dobutamine and other catecholamines. (a) Dopamine; (b) epinephrine; (c) norepinephrine; (d) isoproterenol; (e) dobutamine.

Dobutamine: practical considerations

Indications

- Dynamic exercise is not possible, and
- Contraindication to vasodilator drug.

Contraindications

Absolute contraindications

- Within 1 week of acute myocardial infarction.
- Uncontrolled unstable angina.
- Uncontrolled hypertension (systolic blood pressure ≥200mmHg and/or diastolic blood pressure ≥115mmHg).
- Acute aortic dissection.
- Uncontrolled cardiac dysrhythmias causing symptoms or haemodynamic compromise.

Relative contraindications

- Significant left ventricular outflow tract obstruction (severe aortic stenosis or hypertrophic obstructive cardiomyopathy).

Technical factors arguing against dobutamine

- Left bundle branch block or ventricular pacing (association with imaging artefacts).
- Failure to discontinue β-blocker (limitation of heart rate response).

Dobutamine: performing the stress test

Prior to the test
- β-blockers should be discontinued for five half-lives (typically 48 hours).
- Quick history and possibly examination to exclude contraindications.
- Weigh the patient.
- Explain procedure to the patient, mentioning likely side effects.
- Set up 12-lead ECG monitoring and blood pressure cuff.
- Insert peripheral intravenous cannula with three-way tap.

Protocol
- Dobutamine is available as 20ml vials containing 250mg; draw up 10ml in a 50ml Luer-lock syringe, and dilute to 50ml with 5% dextrose (2.5mg/ml).
- Attach via a giving-set to the three-way tap of the intravenous cannula.
- Record heart rate and blood pressure at baseline.
- Record a 12-lead ECG at baseline.
- Give the dobutamine using an infusion pump as follows, increasing rate until target heart rate is achieved:

10µg/kg/min	3min
20µg/kg/min	3min
30µg/kg/min	3min
40µg/kg/min	3min

- If target heart rate not achieved despite dobutamine 40µg/kg/min for 3 minutes, consider giving up to 4 boluses of atropine 300µg at 1 minute intervals.
- Monitor the 12-lead ECG.
- Record heart rate, blood pressure, and a 12-lead ECG every 2 minutes during the infusion, or if a side effect develops.
- One minute after sustained achievement of the target heart rate, inject the radiopharmaceutical via the three-way tap into the flowing stream of dobutamine (give over 10–20 seconds to avoid pushing in bolus of dobutamine).
- Continue infusion at same level for 1 minute, then stop.

Dobutamine: adverse effects

Minor adverse effects

Around 75% of patients have one or more adverse effects with dobutamine. The most common are:
- Chest pain (31%).
- Palpitation (29%).
- Dizziness and flushing (14%).
- Dyspnoea (14%).
- Headache (14%).

Dysrhythmias

Dobutamine is more dysrhythmogenic than other forms of stress, with significant supraventricular or ventricular tachycardias occurring in 10% of patients. Particular care is necessary in patients known to have severe left ventricular impairment.

Ischaemia

Ischaemic ST segment depression occurs in approximately one-third of patients. Myocardial infarction has occasionally been reported.

Reversal of dobutamine stress with short-acting intravenous β-blockade

Persistent side effects of dobutamine can be reversed by administration of esmolol or metoprolol intravenously. Esmolol is particularly suitable as it has a short half-life, and can be given as a bolus of approximately 50mg.

Radiopharmaceuticals used in myocardial perfusion scintigraphy

General considerations

Any radiopharmaceutical has both chemical and physical properties which determine its physiological and imaging characteristics respectively. Practical considerations such as ease of preparation and cost are also important. Three radiopharmaceuticals are in routine clinical use in myocardial perfusion scintigraphy:

- Thallium-201 (^{201}Tl) as thallous chloride.
- Technetium-99m (^{99m}Tc) sestamibi.
- Technetium-99m (^{99m}Tc) tetrofosmin.

In practice none of these is perfect and each has its own strengths and weaknesses, as summarized below.

Physiological considerations

In myocardial perfusion scintigraphy, the chemical properties of the chosen radiopharmaceutical ensure its uptake by the myocardium in relation to blood flow. The ideal tracer would be entirely extracted from the blood on its first passage through the heart (extraction fraction of 1), leading to a linear relation between absolute perfusion and uptake. In practice, the available perfusion tracers have an extraction fraction significantly lower than 1, which leads to a plateauing of the relation at high perfusion rates (see Fig. 8.1). *Relative* uptake into *hypoperfused* myocardium is thereby overestimated, so the extent and severity of inducible perfusion defects are underestimated. This is a particular concern for the 99mTc-labelled tracers, especially tetrofosmin.

Imaging considerations

Radionuclides emit γ and/or X-ray photons with a characteristic energy and decay half-life. Photon energies of 100–200keV are most suitable for gamma camera imaging: lower energies produce low resolution images with substantial soft tissue attenuation, and electrocardiogram (ECG)-gating is challenging. The half-life determines a patient's effective dose equivalent for a given administered activity: a shorter half-life allows a higher activity to be injected, increasing acquired counts and image quality. In contrast to the physiological considerations, imaging considerations favour the ^{99m}Tc-labelled tracers over ^{201}Tl.

Practical considerations

^{201}Tl must be produced in a commercial cyclotron and delivered to a hospital as required, but is relatively cheap. Sestamibi or tetrofosmin are easily prepared from kits with ^{99m}Tc-pertechnetate eluted from a generator in any hospital radiopharmacy, but tend to be more expensive. ^{99m}Tc-sestamibi is slightly more difficult to work with than ^{99m}Tc-tetrofosmin as it requires boiling in its preparation, whilst image quality can be eroded by poorer gut clearance.

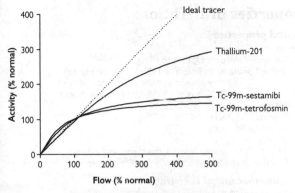

Fig. 8.1 Relationship between absolute myocardial perfusion and tracer uptake for the three radiopharmaceuticals used in myocardial perfusion scintigraphy.

Properties of ^{201}Tl

Physical properties
- Decay:
  - Decays by electron capture to ^{201}Hg.
  - Emitted photons: γ photon at 135keV (3% abundance)
    γ photon at 167keV (10% abundance)
    X-rays at 68–80keV (95% abundance).
- Half-lives:
  - Physical 73.1 hours.
  - Biological 58 hours.
- Dosimetry:
  - Target organs: testes, thyroid, intestines, and kidneys.
  - Effective dose equivalent 14mSv for 80MBq dose.

Radiopharmaceutical preparation
- Delivered as ^{201}Tl from commercial cyclotron.
- ^{203}Pb and ^{202}Tl impurities may be present (<2% activity).
- No in-house preparation required apart from dividing into aliquots.
- No special quality control measures required.
- Dose activity measured pre-injection.

Physiological properties
- Monovalent cation, analogous to potassium.
- Enters myocytes down electrochemical gradient, dependent upon Na^+/K^+-ATPase.
- Myocardial uptake greater than potassium.

After injection (5–15 minutes)
- First-pass myocardial extraction fraction at normal coronary flow rate 0.85.
- Only 5% of injected dose enters myocardium.
- Peak myocardial activity at 5–15 minutes after injection, when only 5% of injected dose remains in blood pool: 'stress' imaging performed at this point.

Redistribution
- ^{201}Tl re-equilibrates between intracellular and extracellular compartments with time, redistributing into all viable myocardium, irrespective of resting perfusion.
- Stress-induced myocardial perfusion defects typically resolve over 3–5 hours.
- Redistribution may be delayed in myocardium subtended by critical epicardial coronary stenosis, taking up to 24 hours.

Excretion
- Excretion is predominantly renal.

^{201}Tl protocols

Stress-redistribution protocol
The standard ^{201}Tl protocol.

Protocol
- ^{201}Tl 80MBq (UK dose) injected during stress.
- Stress image acquisition 5–10 minutes post injection.
- Redistribution acquisition 4 hours post injection.

Practical considerations
- May underestimate viability and hence reversibility of stress defects, as redistribution may be delayed in myocardium subtended by critical coronary stenosis.
- Late redistribution imaging 12–24 hours post injection may overcome the problem, but is inconvenient and image quality is typically poor due to reduced count statistics.

Stress-redistribution-reinjection protocol
This protocol improves detection of myocardial viability and hence reversibility of stress defects.

Protocol
- After redistribution imaging 4 hours post-stress injection, ^{201}Tl 40MBq (UK dose) reinjected at rest.
- Sublingual glyceryl trinitrate 500µg given 5 minutes prior to reinjection may improve resting hypoperfusion and further optimize detection of myocardial viability; beware symptomatic hypotension, particularly in patients not used to taking glyceryl trinitrate therapeutically.
- Resting image acquisition 10–60 minutes after reinjection; may be repeated at 4 and 24 hours to optimize detection of viability, though imaging at 24 hours is inconvenient and yields poor quality acquisitions.

Practical considerations
- Reinjection of ^{201}Tl augments resting blood levels, enhancing redistribution: up to 50% of defects which appear fixed on standard redistribution imaging will reverse following reinjection.
- Not considered routine protocol in most UK centres, though reinjection often performed if severe defect appears fixed using standard stress-redistribution protocol.

Rest-redistribution protocol
Protocol used purely for myocardial viability: no stress test performed so stress-induced hypoperfusion not demonstrated.

Protocol
- ^{201}Tl 80MBq (UK dose) injected at rest.
- Early image acquisition 10–15 minutes after injection to define resting perfusion.
- Delayed acquisition at 3–4 hours to define myocardial viability; may be repeated at 24 hours.

Practical considerations
- Myocardium showing improvement in uptake between the early and late acquisition is likely to be 'hibernating' (viable but with reduced resting perfusion).

Properties of ^{99m}Tc-labelled tracers

Physical properties of ^{99m}Tc

- Decay:
  - Decays by isomeric transition to ^{99}Tc.
  - Emits predominantly γ photons at 140keV.
- Physical half-life 6 hours (biological half-life similar).
- Dosimetry:
  - Target organ: gallbladder.
  - Effective dose equivalent 8–10mSv for 1000MBq of ^{99m}Tc-sestamibi or ^{99m}Tc-tetrofosmin.

Radiopharmaceutical preparation

- ^{99m}Tc produced by β⁻-decay of molybdenum-99 in a commercially available generator.
- Generator eluted daily with sterile 0.9% saline to yield sodium ^{99m}Tc-pertechnetate.
- ^{99m}Tc-pertechnetate added to vial of lyophilized product:
  - Sestamibi (hexakis-2-methoxy-2-methylpropyl-isonitrile): requires boiling for 10 minutes.
  - Tetrofosmin (1,2-bis [bis (2-ethoxyethyl) phosphino] ethane): needs to stand for 15 minutes at room temperature.
- Chromatography performed to ensure purity of radiopharmaceutical.
- Doses drawn from vial and activity calibrated.

Physiological properties

- ^{99m}Tc-sestamibi and ^{99m}Tc-tetrofosmin are lipophilic monovalent cations.
- Passively diffuse across cell and mitochondrial membranes down electrochemical gradient.
- Become fixed within mitochondria with no effective redistribution: myocardial distribution remains static, with clearance only 10–15% at 4 hours.
- First-pass myocardial extraction fraction at normal coronary flow rate: ^{99m}Tc-sestamibi 0.65, ^{99m}Tc-tetrofosmin 0.54; uptake plateaus at lower levels of myocardial perfusion than with ^{201}Tl.
- Only 1–2% of injected dose enters myocardium.
- Rapid clearance from blood pool.

Excretion

- Excretion predominantly via hepatobiliary route.
- Imaging best performed after liver has cleared (usually faster with ^{99m}Tc-tetrofosmin than with ^{99m}Tc-sestamibi).
- Excessive tracer within loops of gut adjacent to heart can impair image quality; gastric activity due to reflux of bile following upper gastrointestinal surgery can be particularly problematic.

- Gut activity less of a problem following tracer injection during exercise compared with pharmacological stress or rest due to splanchnic vasoconstriction.
- Variety of foods and drinks may be given between injection and imaging as aids to clearance, and most departments have preferred protocol: milk, chocolate, and fatty foods encourage gallbladder contraction; carbonated drinks may inflate stomach and push 'hot' gut loops down and away from heart.

^{99m}Tc-sestamibi and ^{99m}Tc-tetrofosmin protocols

Two-day protocol
Optimal protocol from a technical viewpoint as identical tracer dose used for stress and resting parts of study.
- ^{99m}Tc-sestamibi or ^{99m}Tc-tetrofosmin 400MBq (UK dose) injected during stress.
- Stress acquisition 30–60 minutes post injection (depending on tracer and mode of stress).
- At second visit >24 hours (preferably >48 hours) later, similar dose injected at rest.
- Resting acquisition performed 45–90 minutes later (depending on tracer).
- May omit resting part of study if stress acquisition unequivocally normal.

One-day protocols
- Only one visit required, so may be more practical than 2-day protocol for frail patients or those travelling long distances.
- Small dose of tracer given for first part of study, followed a few hours later by higher (at least three-fold) dose for second part to swamp any residual myocardial activity.
- Potential problems:
  - Suboptimal quality of first low-dose acquisition.
  - Inadequate swamping effect of high dose.

One-day stress-rest protocol
Commonest 1-day protocol used in the UK.

Protocol
- ^{99m}Tc-sestamibi or ^{99m}Tc-tetrofosmin 250MBq (UK dose) injected during stress.
- Stress acquisition 30–60 minutes post injection (depending on tracer and mode of stress).
- 3–4 hours after stress injection, ^{99m}Tc-sestamibi or ^{99m}Tc-tetrofosmin 750MBq (UK dose) injected at rest.
- Resting acquisition performed 45–90 minutes later (depending on tracer).
- May omit resting part of study if stress acquisition unequivocally normal, so this protocol most suitable for patients with low-likelihood of disease and no history of myocardial infarction.

Practical considerations
Stress-rest order may underestimate defect reversibility, particularly if inadequate delay between injections:
- Stress-induced hypoperfusion may not have fully resolved.
- Absolute myocardial perfusion higher during stress than at rest, so proportion of dose taken up by myocardium is higher following the smaller stress injection than following the higher resting injection; this would tend to undermine the swamping effect.

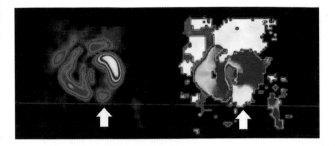

Fig. 5.3 Amplitude (left) and phase (right) images of left ventricular aneurysm (white arrow), which has amplitude but is 180° out of phase with the rest of the ventricle.

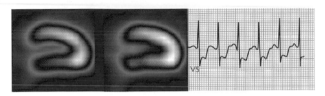

Fig. 7.3 Exercise test may aid reporting. This 62 year old man underwent a one-day exercise-rest ^{99m}Tc-tetrosfosmin SPECT study. This demonstrated an equivocal reversible inferior perfusion defect which could easily have been dismissed as attenuation artefact (left panel shows representative vertical long axis slice, stress on left, rest on right). However the exercise test was strongly positive with limiting chest pain and deep ST depression at only 4 minutes of the Bruce protocol (right panel). Subsequent coronary angiography demonstrated a severe right coronary artery stenosis.

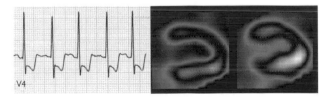

Fig. 7.8 Ischaemic ECG during an adenosine infusion (left panel). The patient was subsequently found to have a high-risk perfusion study (transient ischaemic dilatation and large reversible anteroapical perfusion defect, right panel), with severe multivessel coronary disease at angiography.

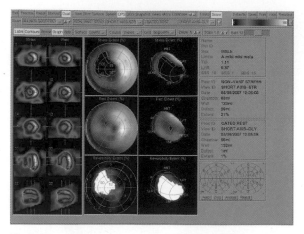

Fig. 9.4 Quantitative analysis from commercially available software package for patient with reversible anteroapical and septal perfusion defect. Left panel: short axis (apical, mid and basal), horizontal long axis and vertical long axis slices for stress (left) and rest (right). Middle left panel: stress (top), rest (middle) and reversibility (bottom) polar plots, with calculated defect extent overlaid in black. Middle right panel: stress (top), rest (middle) and reversibility (bottom) three-dimensional renderings, with calculated defect extent overlaid in black. Right panel: semi-quantitative and quantitative indices.

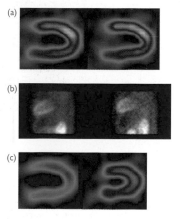

Fig. 9.5 Inferior attenuation artefact. (a) Vertical long axis slice (stress left, rest right) showing reduced counts inferiorly. (b) Raw data projection (stress left, rest right) shows diaphragm overlying inferior wall. (c) Gated resting slice (end-diastole left, end-systole right) shows thickening and movement of inferior wall.

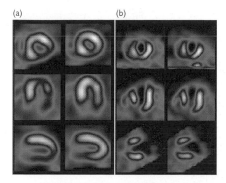

Fig. 9.7 Reversible inferolateral perfusion defect (a) and fixed apical perfusion defect (b). Left column stress, right column rest; top to bottom: short axis, horizontal long axis, vertical long axis.

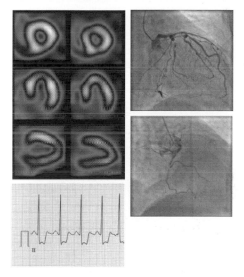

Fig. 9.8 Balanced multivessel coronary disease. A 76-year-old lady presented with a recent increase in her longstanding chest pain. SPECT slices (top left) demonstrated no definite perfusion defect, but there was (1) transient ischaemic dilatation of the left ventricular cavity with prominence of the right ventricular free wall; (2) a strongly positive exercise test, with limiting chest pain and deep ST depression at only 2 minutes 16 seconds of the modified Bruce protocol (bottom left). Subsequent coronary angiography demonstrated severe proximal three vessel coronary disease (right).

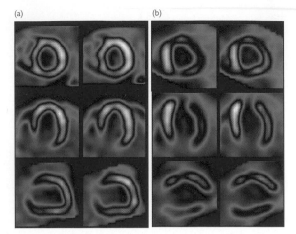

Fig. 9.9 Perfusion studies of two patients presenting with heart failure but no definite history of coronary disease or chest pain. (a) Dilated globular left ventricular cavity, with no perfusion abnormality; appearances typical of dilated cardiomyopathy. (b) Dilated left ventricular cavity, fixed apical perfusion defect, reversible lateral perfusion defect, possible inferior perfusion defect though attenuation likely; appearances strongly suggestive of ischaemic left ventricular dysfunction. Left column stress, right column rest; top short axis slice, middle horizontal long axis slice, bottom vertical long axis slice.

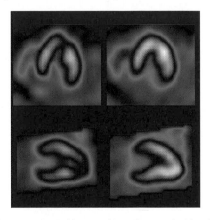

Fig. 9.10 Appearance in apical hypertrophic cardiomyopathy. Note the prominent apex on the rest acquisition, with an inducible apical perfusion abnormality during exercise. Left column stress, right column rest; top row horizontal long axis slice, bottom row vertical long axis slice.

One-day rest-stress protocol
Commonest 1-day protocol used in the USA.

Protocol
- ^{99m}Tc-sestamibi or ^{99m}Tc-tetrofosmin 250MBq (UK dose) injected at rest.
- Resting acquisition 45–90 minutes post injection (depending on tracer).
- ^{99m}Tc-sestamibi or ^{99m}Tc-tetrofosmin 750MBq (UK dose) injected during stress: can follow immediately after resting acquisition.
- Stress acquisition performed 30–60 minutes later (depending on tracer and mode of stress).

Practical considerations
Rest-stress order may underestimate extent and severity of reversible hypoperfusion due to residual counts from resting study contaminating stress acquisition.

Augmentation of resting study with glyceryl trinitrate for viability assessment

- In order to maximize tracer uptake into viable myocardium, particularly if subtended by critical epicardial coronary stenosis, sublingual glyceryl trinitrate (500µg) may be administered 5 minutes prior to the resting injection.
- Symptomatic hypotension should be anticipated, particularly in patients not used to taking glyceryl trinitrate therapeutically.
- Nitrate augmentation mandatory if ^{99m}Tc protocol being used to identify hibernating myocardium; also advisable in any patient who has (or might have) stress perfusion defect, to optimize assessment of viability and hence reversibility.

Dual isotope (rest ^{201}Tl / stress ^{99m}Tc) imaging

Combines advantages of rest ^{201}Tl for viability and stress ^{99m}Tc in a time-efficient protocol. Popular in certain US centres, but seldom used in the UK. Lower photon energy of ^{201}Tl (68–80keV) does not interfere with higher energy window used for ^{99m}Tc imaging (140keV).

Protocol
- ^{201}Tl 40–80MBq injected at rest; image acquisition at 30 minutes.
- Stress can be performed immediately afterwards, with injection of ^{99m}Tc-sestamibi or ^{99m}Tc-tetrofosmin 400–750MBq; image acquisition at 30–60 minutes.

Practical considerations
May be difficult to assess reversibility given that stress and resting images derived from different radionuclides.

Other perfusion tracers not in current clinical use

^{99m}Tc-teboroxime

- Highly lipophilic, neutral charge.
- Preparation similar to ^{99m}Tc-sestamibi.
- Myocardial uptake is independent of metabolic activity.
- First-pass extraction fraction even higher than ^{201}Tl, with linear relation to myocardial perfusion throughout physiological range.
- Imaging technically difficult due to poor myocardial retention:
  - Excellent images at 1–2 minutes.
  - Rapid bi-exponential washout (68% with half-time 2 minutes, 32% with half-time 78 minutes).
- Hepatic excretion.
- Developments in ultra-fast image acquisition using multi-headed gamma cameras might allow ^{99m}Tc-teboroxime to be used in routine clinical practice.

^{99m}Tc-N-NOET

- ^{99m}Tc-bis[N-ethoxy, N-ethyl dithiocarbamato] nitrido.
- No longer being developed, but formerly the newest ^{99m}Tc agent.
- Lipophilic, neutral charge.
- Good perfusion tracer with extraction fraction similar to ^{99m}Tc-teboroxime, but longer myocardial retention.
- Good viability tracer with significant redistribution, as with ^{201}Tl.
- High lung uptake due to solubilizing agent (cyclodextrin).
- Quality control and image quality were occasionally problematic.
- Phase III trials showed promise, but product was never licensed for clinical use.

Myocardial perfusion scintigraphy: image interpretation

Planar acquisitions

Introduction

Planar acquisition has been largely superseded by single photon emission computed tomography (SPECT), which allows left ventricular (LV) myocardial perfusion to be viewed as sets of orthogonal slices familiar to cardiologists from other imaging modalities. SPECT also offers improved diagnostic sensitivity, particularly in single-vessel coronary disease. Nevertheless, planar imaging actually provides better spatial resolution than SPECT as the camera head can be brought in closer to the heart. It should also be remembered that the original literature demonstrating the excellent diagnostic and prognostic power of myocardial perfusion scintigraphy was based on planar imaging. Planar imaging is still useful in occasional patients, for example those unable to lie flat for SPECT who require upright imaging.

Practical considerations

- Images are acquired in three standard projections (see Fig. 9.1):
  - Anterior.
  - 45° left anterior oblique.
  - Left lateral.
- Confirmation of adequate image quality should be performed before the patient leaves the department.
- Image interpretation should be performed using greyscale on the computer workstation.
- Artefacts are a particular issue and repeat imaging may be required.

Image interpretation

- Extracardiac tracer uptake:
  - Excessive uptake in the liver or gallbladder may be problematic.
  - Focal uptake in the breast, lung, or thyroid may represent malignancy.
- Lung uptake (primarily with ^{201}Tl):
  - Lung : heart ratio should be calculated: in anterior projection, place regions of interest around the right lung field and the heart.
  - Upper limit of normal is typically 0.8.
  - Increase suggests chronically or transiently elevated left atrial pressure (i.e. LV dysfunction) and is associated with high risk.
- LV cavity size:
  - Dilatation on both stress and rest images suggests significant resting systolic dysfunction.
  - Reversible dilatation on stress image only [transient ischaemic dilatation (TID)] suggests large ischaemic burden.
- Appearance of right ventricle:
  - Dilated cavity suggests dysfunction.
  - Count density of free wall normally 50% that of LV myocardium
  - Increase on both stress and rest images suggests right ventricular hypertrophy.
  - Reversible increase on stress image only may indicate global hypoperfusion of *LV* myocardium.

- Regional myocardial perfusion on stress and rest images:
  - Defect severity: mild, moderate, or severe.
  - Defect extent: small, medium, or large.
  - Defect reversibility: fixed, partial reversibility, complete reversibility.
  - If required, semi-quantitative analysis using a 15-segment model can be performed: each segment is scored for severity of count reduction, and the values summed for stress and rest acquisitions (Fig. 9.1 and Table 9.1).
- Quantitative analysis using background subtraction may be used:
  - Images compared with tracer-specific and gender-specific normal database for local population: pixels with counts more than two standard deviations below normal are considered abnormal.
  - May improve reporting confidence, especially for inexperienced readers.
  - Should be regarded as an aid, but is no substitute for visual analysis.

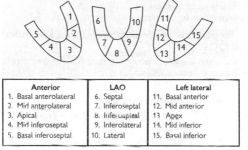

Anterior	LAO	Left lateral
1. Basal anterolateral	6. Septal	11. Basal anterior
2. Mid anterolateral	7. Inferoseptal	12. Mid anterior
3. Apical	8. Inferoapical	13. Apex
4. Mid inferoseptal	9. Inferolateral	14. Mid inferior
5. Basal inferoseptal	10. Lateral	15. Basal inferior

Fig. 9.1 Planar imaging segments.

Table 9.1 Semi-quantitative scoring

Score	Category	Count density
0	Normal perfusion	70–100%
1	Mild reduction in counts	50–70%
2	Moderate reduction in counts	30–50%
3	Severe reduction in counts	10–30%
4	Absent counts	0–10%

General approach to reporting SPECT images

A methodical approach should be taken to ensure consistency and accuracy. Good quality control (QC) through audit is then easy to achieve. The aim is to integrate all available data to produce a report which is both accurate and clinically useful. The following approach is suggested:

Read the referral letter carefully

- Note previous cardiac history or investigations.
- Understand indication for myocardial perfusion scintigraphy.
- Identify specific clinical questions.

Check patient identifying details against details on workstation images

Scrutinize stress test data

- Note method of stress.
- Confirm adequacy of stress.
- Document stress test results.

Review looped cine of raw data projections and other relevant QC tools

- Consider issues likely to produce artefacts in processed slices.
- Identify cardiac abnormalities.
- Identify non-cardiac pathology.

Check performance of quantitation software (e.g. accuracy of myocardial contouring) and attenuation correction (AC) if used

Study processed tomographic slices in all three planes

- Check stress and rest slices correspond accurately.
- Qualitative assessment.
- Semi-quantitative scoring.
- Quantitative analysis.
- Identify possible artefacts.

Study gated images

- Regional function: thickening and movement.
- Global function: volumes and ejection fraction.

Reach a firm conclusion and answer the clinical question

Review looped cine of raw data projections

This is probably the most important QC procedure. It should be done immediately after the acquisition, again during image processing, and once more during formal reporting. The cine of the raw data displays each of the planar projections acquired as the heads of the gamma camera orbit the patient, animated as a cine loop. It should be displayed in greyscale. If a dual-headed camera is used, half the projections will be acquired on one head, and half on the other, with a transition halfway through the cine. A number of features should be noted.

Issues likely to produce artefacts in processed slices

Poor count statistics

Poor count statistics in all projections suggests:
- Inadequate tracer dose.
- Extravasation of dose.
- Inadequate acquisition time per projection.

Loss of counts on only certain projections in a gated acquisition can indicate excessive beat rejection during those projections.

Heart not completely in field of view in some projections

In obese patients, the apex may be 'cut-off' in certain projections if the acquisition has been carelessly set up.

Patient motion

The heart should appear to rotate smoothly from projection to projection without jumps in any direction.

Sudden patient movement is seen as an abrupt jump on equivalent projections from each camera head.

More gradual progressive movement during an acquisition may be poorly appreciated from projection to projection, but produces an abrupt jump from the final projection on the first head to the first projection on the second head.

The sinogram may also help to identify patient movement. This is a static image representing a single transaxial level, with corresponding rows of pixels from successive planar projections stacked on top of each.

Excessive bowel activity

Note poor clearance of tracer from the liver and gallbladder, or 'hot' loops of bowel or occasionally stomach adjacent to the heart.

Attenuating structures

Note prominent photopaenic structures passing in front of the heart:
- Breasts and breast implants in women.
- Diaphragm in men.
- Metal objects (e.g. pacemaker box, coins, nitrate spray in top pocket).

Cardiac abnormalities

Perfusion defects

Perfusion defects are sometimes obvious on the raw data cine.

Dilated LV cavity

Dilatation on both stress and rest images suggests resting dysfunction.

Reversible dilatation seen on stress image only [transient ischaemic dilatation (TID)] suggests large ischaemic burden.

Appearance of the right ventricle

Cavity dilatation may indicate dysfunction.

Increased count density in free wall on:
- Both stress and rest images suggests right ventricular hypertrophy.
- On stress image only may indicate global hypoperfusion of *LV* myocardium.

Increased lung uptake of tracer

Increased lung uptake of tracer, especially with ^{201}Tl, suggests chronically or transiently impaired LV function.

Non-cardiac uptake of tracer

Subcutaneous extravasation in the arm of all or part of the tracer injection may be visualized, and may explain poor count statistics within the heart.

Uptake in axillary lymph nodes does not necessarily indicate pathology, and is usually due to lymphatic drainage of extravasated tracer.

Focal uptake in the breast, lung, or thyroid can indicate malignancy.

Qualitative and semi-quantitative evaluation of tomographic slices

Display

By convention, reconstructed and reorientated SPECT slices are displayed in rows in the three standard orthogonal planes, with corresponding stress slices placed above rest slices:

* Short axis from apex (left) to base (right).
* Vertical long axis from septum (left) to lateral wall (right).
* Horizontal long axis from inferior wall (left) to anterior wall (right).

Count density in each pixel is coded according to a colour scale, relative to the pixel of maximal counts within the myocardium. A continuous colour scale (e.g. grey or 'GE cool') is preferable to a discontinuous one (e.g. rainbow), so that small changes in count density between pixels cannot produce abrupt changes in colour with the false appearance of a perfusion defect.

Qualitative assessment

* Ensure stress and rest slices are correctly orientated and aligned.
* Examine stress slices, identifying the location, extent and severity of regions of reduced count density from most severe to least severe.
* Examine rest slices, identifying location and completeness of any improvement, or paradoxical worsening.
* In everyday clinical practice, when full semi-quantitative analysis is unnecessary, a simplified 9-segment model of the LV myocardium can be used to give a simple description of defect extent (one segment for the apex, and a basal and mid segment for each for the anterior, lateral, inferior, and septal walls).

Semi-quantitative assessment

A number of different models have been used to segment the LV myocardium. In an attempt to achieve uniformity across different imaging modalities, and using post-mortem studies to ensure that segments corresponds to an equivalent mass of myocardium, a 17-segment model is currently advocated by the American Society of Nuclear Cardiology and other American bodies[1]. This is similar to the 16-segment model commonly used in echocardiography, but adds an 'apical cap' (Fig. 9.2).

Each segment can be scored for perfusion on a five-point scale (Table 9.2). A segment with reduced count density on the stress acquisition is considered reversible if it improves to grade 0 or 1, and/or there is a ≥2 grade improvement.

Defect extent can be categorized according to the percentage of the overall LV myocardium involved (Table 9.3).

The summed score for all segments can be used as an index of overall abnormality for both stress (summed stress score, SSS) and rest (summed rest score, SRS) acquisitions. The difference between SSS and SRS, the summed difference score (SDS), is an index of overall reversible hypoperfusion.

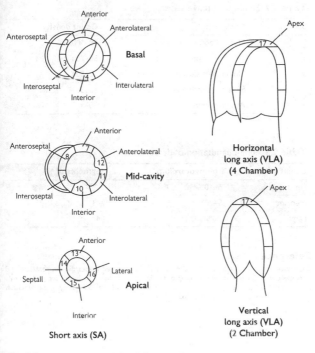

Fig. 9.2 17-Segment model of the left ventricular myocardium, reproduced with permission.[1]

Table 9.2 Semi-quantitative scoring

Score	Category	Count density
0	Normal perfusion	70–100%
1	Mild reduction in counts	50–70%
2	Moderate reduction in counts	30–50%
3	Severe reduction in counts	10–30%
4	Absent counts	0–10%

Table 9.3 Semi-quantitation of defect extent

Extent	% of myocardium	Segments of 17
Small	5–10%	1–2
Medium	15–20%	2–3
Large	>20%	≥4

References

1 Cerqueira MD, Weissman NJ, Dilsizian V, *et al*. Standardized myocardial segmentation and nomenclature for tomographic imaging of the heart: a statement for healthcare professionals from the Cardiac Imaging Committee of the Council on Clinical Cardiology of the American Heart Association. *Circulation* 2002; **105**: 539–42.

Quantitative analysis

SPECT provides information about relative myocardial perfusion, and unlike positron emission tomography (PET) cannot be used to calculate absolute myocardial perfusion. In the context of SPECT, 'quantitative analysis' therefore refers to the use of sophisticated software to compare an acquisition with a database of normal studies, thereby generating values for the extent and severity of defects.

Polar or 'bullseye' plots

A circular polar plot is used to summarize a processed SPECT acquisition. It is generated from the reconstructed and reorientated short axis slices (or occasionally radial long axis slices). With appropriate scaling, short axis slices are arranged concentrically from the apex at the centre to the base at the circumference.

The 'raw' polar plot can aid visual appreciation of the topology of a complex defect, but also allows comparison with a normal database.

A 17-segment grid can be superimposed on the polar plot, and the mean percentage counts displayed in each segment (see Fig. 9.3). Comparison with a normal database can be used to assign a semi-quantitative severity score automatically.

Quantified polar plots can be generated which display only abnormal pixels (Fig. 9.4). These are usually defined as having percentage counts below the lower 95% confidence limit for the corresponding pixel in a normal database. Defect extent can be expressed as a proportion of the overall LV myocardium.

Stress and rest plots can be compared, and the degree of reversibility of defects displayed on another plot.

Normal databases

Normal databases should be derived from patients with a low pre-test probability of coronary disease. Databases of patients with normal coronary angiography or asymptomatic volunteers may not be representative of the patient population to be studied. Any 'normal' database will include patients who in reality have mild perfusion abnormalities, with the potential for error.

For optimal quantitative analysis, normal databases should be specific for:
• Radiopharmaceutical and protocol.
• Local patient population.
• Gender.

Sensitivity and specificity of quantitative analysis

The rules used to define abnormality in relation to a normal database are arbitrary, but set the sensitivity and specificity of the software for identifying real perfusion defects. The threshold for abnormality can be adjusted according to reader preference. A high threshold produces good specificity at the expense of sensitivity, but the reader is required to look carefully for subtle defects that the software will miss. Quantitative analysis should be used to bolster reporting confidence, particularly that of inexperienced readers, but should not be used to 'overrule' the qualitative assessment of SPECT slices.

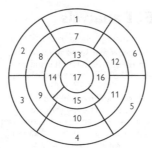

1. Basal anterior   7. Mid anterior   13. Apical anterior
2. Basal anteroseptal   8. Mid anteroseptal   14. Apical septal
3. Basal inferoseptal   9. Mid inferoseptal   15. Apical inferior
4. Basal inferior   10. Mid inferior   16. Apical lateral
5. Basal inferolateral   11. Mid inferolateral   17. Apex
6. Basal anterolateral   12. Mid anterolateral

Fig. 9.3 17-Segment grid for polar plot of the left ventricular myocardium.

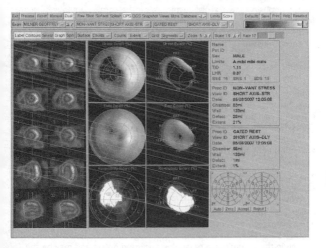

Fig. 9.4 Quantitative analysis from commercially available software package for patient with reversible anteroapical and septal perfusion defect. Left panel: short axis (apical, mid and basal), horizontal long axis and vertical long axis slices for stress (left) and rest (right). Middle left panel: stress (top), rest (middle) and reversibility (bottom) polar plots, with calculated defect extent overlaid in black. Middle right panel: stress (top), rest (middle) and reversibility (bottom) three-dimensional renderings, with calculated defect extent overlaid in black. Right panel: semi-quantitative and quantitative indices. (See also colour plate section.)

Gated SPECT

Display

- View cine loops of short axis slices at apical, mid, and basal levels, together with representative horizontal and vertical long axis slices.
- Normalize pixels to the pixel of maximal counts in the end-systolic frame.
- Use greyscale to assess wall motion, and continuous colour scale (e.g. 'GE cool') to assess thickening (brightening).
- Use quantitative software to apply endocardial and epicardial contours, aiding the assessment of wall motion and allowing calculation of global indices; visually check accuracy of contours.

Regional wall motion and thickening

Inward motion of the myocardium in systole can be visually appreciated. Myocardial thickening from diastole to systole lies below the spatial resolution of SPECT and cannot be directly assessed. However, the count density of normally functioning myocardium appears to increase in systole due to the partial volume effect, and this brightening can be used as a surrogate for thickening.

As for perfusion, myocardial segments can be semi-quantitatively scored for function using a six-point scale (see Table 9.4). In practice, the distinction between degrees of hypokinesia is difficult, whilst dyskinesia of an aneurysm is seldom appreciated due to its severely reduced or absent tracer uptake, so the scale can be simplified to normal, hypokinesia and akinesia. Summed motion or summed thickening scores can be calculated, analogous to summed perfusion scores.

When interpreting regional function on gated SPECT, normal variants must be borne in mind:

- Lateral wall appears more vigorous than septum, especially at the base.
- Basal segments appear relatively hypokinetic approaching the mitral annulus.
- In left bundle branch block (LBBB), the septum may move paradoxically.

The assessment of regional function should be used to inform the perfusion findings:

- A 'fixed perfusion defect' with normal wall motion may represent artefact rather than scar.
- An inducible wall motion abnormality seen only on the post-stress study may reflect post-ischaemic stunning; occasionally this occurs even in the absence of a reversible perfusion defect and may be the only clue to underlying ischaemia.

Global LV volumes and ejection fraction

Modern quantitative software automatically calculates LV end-systolic and end-diastolic volumes and ejection fraction. These programs have been extensively validated against contrast X-ray ventriculography, radionuclide ventriculography, or cardiac magnetic resonance imaging. In general the values are accurate and reproducible, but their validity should be confirmed visually: algorithms attempt to model the LV to a predefined shape, and this may not be valid if, for example, there is a severe and extensive perfusion defect with aneurysm formation.

If, as is commonly done, gating is performed using only 8 frames, ejection fraction tends to be underestimated by 3–4 points due to suboptimal temporal resolution of the time–volume curve with overestimation of end-systolic volume: this is easily overcome by using 16 frames.

Gated SPECT LV ejection fraction is most accurate in the low to mid range of values. At high values there is a tendency to overestimation due to the limited spatial resolution of SPECT, with underestimation of cavity size in small ventricles, particularly at end-systole. Very high values (>70%) for ejection fraction should not be quoted in the final report in case they are taken to imply abnormal hyperdynamic function, and LV function is best described qualitatively as 'normal'.

Volumes and ejection fraction are valuable when comparing serial gated SPECT studies. As with any imaging technique, caution should be exercised when comparing values with other modalities, such as echocardiography or cardiac magnetic resonance imaging.

Table 9.4 Semi-quantitative scale for wall motion and thickening on gated SPECT

Category	Score
Normokinesia	0
Mild hypokinesia	1
Moderate hypokinesia	2
Severe hypokinesia	3
Akinesia	4
Dyskinesia	5

Attenuation correction

In the majority of studies it is possible to identify attenuation artefacts with a high degree of confidence by inspecting the looped cine of the raw data and gated SPECT images, together with quantitative analysis. However even very experienced reporters are unable to distinguish between real defects and attenuation in all cases. To provide additional help, attenuation correction (AC) techniques are becoming increasingly routine. AC appears to reduce the number of equivocal reports, and allows a higher proportion of patients with a normal stress study to be confidently identified as such without the need for rest imaging.

Using AC in reporting

Non-AC and AC images should both be viewed during reporting. The overall clinical setting should always be borne in mind before changing a report based on AC images.

A normal attenuation corrected study usually demonstrates uniform count density in all regions apart from the apex and apical anterior wall, which appear relatively photopaenic. This is exaggerated in large hearts, especially in men. The unsuspecting observer might therefore report a spurious perfusion defect in the territory of the left anterior descending (LAD) artery.

AC may create its own new artefacts, for example, subdiaphragmatic tracer activity may be exaggerated, with artefactually reduced count density in the heart.

Image artefacts

Image artefacts are relatively common in both planar and SPECT acquisitions, and can make an otherwise normal study appear abnormal, particularly to the inexperienced reader. Some artefacts can be prevented entirely by careful attention to detail in gamma camera QC and image acquisition and processing. Others are unavoidable in certain patients, but can usually be anticipated and recognized as long as the reader has a good understanding of the technical aspects of myocardial perfusion scintigraphy. The presence of an artefact should be recognized in the final report, especially if any technical correction has been used in the processing, but every effort should be made to avoid equivocation as to the study's normality.

Image artefacts can be classified as follows:

Instrumentation-related artefacts

- Non-uniformity of the flood field.
- Centre of rotation errors.
- Excessive patient-to-detector distance.
- Apex excluded from field of view in some projections.

Processing-related and display-related artefacts

- Excessive bowel activity.
- Incorrect reorientation and slice alignment.
- Discontinuous colour scale.

Patient-related artefacts

- Motion of patient during image acquisition.
- Anterior soft tissue (breast) attenuation.
- Inferior (diaphragmatic) attenuation.
- Diffuse soft tissue attenuation.
- Attenuation by non-anatomical structures.
- Normal variants giving the appearance of a perfusion abnormality.

Gating artefact

Instrumentation-related artefacts

Compared with other types of medical imaging equipment, gamma cameras are potentially unstable and require a programme of regular careful QC checks by technical staff and medical physicists. A log of all these checks and any corrections is mandatory, as is regular servicing by a qualified engineer. Some malfunctions can occur abruptly during the course of a day's scanning (e.g. failure of a photomultiplier tube). Fortunately, most are gradual and can usually be identified from QC checks before they have reached a level at which they could affect patient studies. Instrumentation errors tend to produce similar artefacts in consecutive patient studies, helping to identify the cause.

Non-uniformity of the flood field

Cause

- Occurs with defects in collimators, crystal, photomultiplier tubes, or camera electronics.

Appearance

- Produces photon-deficient ring artefacts in the reconstructed SPECT images.
- May cause an apparent perfusion defect where a ring crosses the myocardium.

Prevention

- Usually detected by daily 'floods' performed as part of camera QC.

Recognition

- Inspection of raw data planar images may help identify the problem.

Centre of rotation errors

Cause

- Incorrect centre of rotation prevents accurate back-projection of SPECT data.
- Abnormal angulation of camera head may cause similar problems.

Appearance

- Gives appearance of shifting of a myocardial wall on reconstructed SPECT images.
- May give the appearance of perfusion defect(s) at the point(s) of shifting.

Prevention

- Regular QC checks of centre of rotation and head alignment should minimize the risk.

Recognition

- Suspect if present in consecutive studies.

Excessive patient-to-detector distance

- With a parallel-hole collimator, resolution falls with increasing distance between patient and camera head.

Apex excluded from field of view in some projections

Cause

- In obese patients, unless care is taken defining the orbit it is possible for the apex of the heart to be 'cut-off' at the edge of the field of view in certain projections.

Appearance

- Can give appearance of apical defect.

Recognition

- Problem should be identifiable from looped cine of raw data projections.

Processing-related and display-related artefacts

Excessive bowel activity

Cause

- Excessive bowel activity may be a particular problem when ^{99m}Tc-sestamibi or ^{99m}Tc-tetrofosmin is used.
- ^{99m}Tc- labelled tracers localize in the liver, pass into the gallbladder, and then enter the small bowel (or occasionally the stomach if there is reflux of bile).

Appearance

- Visceral activity overlying the inferior wall may obscure a real inferior perfusion defect.
- Normalization to high visceral activity overlying the inferior wall may create relative apparent defects in the other walls.
- High visceral activity adjacent to the heart may cause an artefactual reduction in counts in the inferior wall when filtered back projection is used ('ramp filter artefact').

Prevention

- Can be reduced by using exercise stress whenever possible, even if submaximal and in combination with a vasodilator drug.
- Food (fatty, to promote gallbladder contraction) and drink (water or milk) may improve clearance.
- Carbonated drinks (to inflate stomach and push away gut loops) and lemon juice (to promote biliary excretion into the gallbladder without gallbladder contraction) are also used.
- Adequate time should be left prior to imaging following injection of ^{99m}Tc-sestamibi and, to a lesser extent, ^{99m}Tc-tetrofosmin, particularly after vasodilator stress.
- If gut clearance poor on initial acquisition, consider repeating after a further delay with additional food and drink.
- Use of iterative reconstruction rather than filtered back projection avoids the 'ramp filter artefact'.

Recognition

- Excessive gut activity is easily identified on cine of raw data planar images.

Incorrect reorientation and slice alignment

- Inaccurate reorientation of the reconstructed slices to the long axes of the LV may lead to uncertainty regarding the location of a defect.
- Differences in reorientation or incorrect slice alignment between stress and rest acquisitions can cause errors in the assessment of defect reversibility.
- Routine inspection of the reoriented stress and rest slices alongside each other should identify a problem and allow adjustment.

Discontinuous colour scale

- When slices are displayed using a discontinuous colour scale (e.g. rainbow), small changes in count density between pixels can sometimes produce abrupt changes in colour, giving the appearance of a perfusion defect.
- Continuous colour scales (e.g. greyscale or 'GE cool') avoid this problem.

Patient-related artefacts (1)

A number of patient-related factors can introduce apparent inhomogeneities into processed SPECT images, giving the appearance of perfusion defects. Whilst some of these artefacts can be avoided by careful patient preparation and where necessary repeating the acquisition, attenuation artefacts are related to body habitus and must simply be recognized for what they are. Careful inspection of the looped cine of raw data projections may be of value in the identification of attenuation artefacts, as are gated and attenuation-corrected images where available.

Motion of patient during image acquisition

Cause

- Common source of image artefact.
- Patients can move in vertical, lateral or rotational directions.
- Heart may move gradually upwards ('upward creep') during the immediate post-exercise acquisition of a ^{201}Tl study as lung volume progressively falls.

Appearance

- Excessive movement during image acquisition may cause shift of myocardial wall on reconstructed SPECT images.
- May give the appearance of perfusion defect(s) at the point(s) of shifting, with 'streaming' away from the edge.

Prevention

- Less of a problem with multi-headed cameras as acquisition time is reduced.
- Movement may be reduced by careful patient explanation, comfortable posture during image acquisition, strapping, and quiet environment in camera room.
- If a ^{99m}Tc-labelled tracer has been used, and the patient is likely to do better the second time, image acquisition should be repeated if excessive movement is present.
- If repeating the acquisition is inappropriate, validated software may be used to correct for vertical movement (motion-corrected cine of raw data and sinogram should be checked to ensure success).

Recognition

- Inspection of looped cine of raw data projections and sinogram should identify significant patient movement.
- Abrupt movement is seen on single corresponding projection from each camera head.
- Gradual movement throughout the acquisition (e.g. as the patient relaxes) is seen as a step between the final projection from the first head and the first projection from the second head.

Patient-related artefacts (2)

Anterior soft tissue (breast) attenuation

Cause
- Important source of artefact in women.
- Inexact correlation between breast size and degree of attenuation.

Appearance
- Appearance of perfusion defect variably affecting anterior or lateral wall.
- Usually fixed 'defect', but may be more prominent on low-dose acquisition of 1-day ^{99m}Tc protocol producing apparent reversibility.

Prevention
- Image with brassiere off, possibly with strapping, but essential that breast position is identical on stress and rest acquisitions to avoid spurious reversibility.

Recognition
- Photopaenic breast shadows passing in front of heart on looped cine of raw data projections.
- Normal wall motion and thickening on gated SPECT.
- Removal of the 'defect' by AC.

Inferior (diaphragmatic) attenuation (Fig. 9.5, p. 148)

Cause
- Important source of artefact, usually in men.
- Particularly occurs in obese patients or those with a dilated LV.

Appearance
- Appearance of inferior perfusion defect.
- Usually fixed 'defect', but may be more prominent on low-dose acquisition of 1-day ^{99m}Tc protocol producing apparent reversibility.

Prevention
- May be reduced by prone imaging; upright imaging has also been suggested.

Recognition
- Photopaenic diaphragmatic shadow passing in front of inferior wall on looped cine of raw data projections.
- Normal wall motion and thickening on gated SPECT.
- Removal of the 'defect' by AC.

Diffuse soft tissue attenuation

Cause
- Sometimes affects obese patients.
- Entire myocardium attenuated, but more distant regions (i.e. basal segments) more affected.

Appearance
- Appearance of reduced count density affecting all basal segments of the LV myocardium.

Recognition
- Non-coronary distribution of apparent defect.
- Normal wall motion and thickening on gated SPECT.
- Removal of the 'defect' by AC.

Attenuation by non-anatomical structures

Cause
- Affects patients with breast implants, pacemakers, metal objects in top pocket (e.g. coins or nitrate spray).

Appearance
- Appearance of anterior perfusion defect.
- Usually fixed 'defect', assuming that attenuating object not removed between acquisitions.

Prevention
- Check shirt pockets for removable objects prior to image acquisition, repeat acquisition if missed.

Recognition
- Photopaenic shadow passing in front of heart on raw data cine.
- Normal wall motion and thickening on gated SPECT.

Cardiac variants giving the appearance of a perfusion abnormality

Short septum
- The basal portion of the interventricular septum is membranous and does not take up tracer, so the septum appears shorter than the other LV walls.
- This can be misinterpreted as a fixed basal septal perfusion defect by an inexperienced reporter.

Apical 'thinning'
- The apical myocardium can appear thinner than that of the other LV walls, giving the appearance of a fixed perfusion defect.
- Clue is small size of the defect, with normal contraction on gated SPECT.

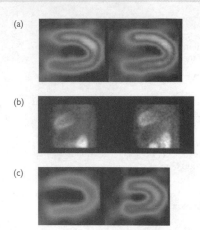

Fig. 9.5 Inferior attenuation artefact. (a) Vertical long axis slice (stress left, rest right) showing reduced counts inferiorly. (b) Raw data projection (stress left, rest right) shows diaphragm overlying inferior wall. (c) Gated resting slice (end-diastole left, end-systole right) shows thickening and movement of inferior wall. (See also colour plate section.)

Gating artefact

Cause
- During a gated SPECT acquisition, significant variation in R-R interval (e.g. in atrial fibrillation or frequent ectopy) can lead to rejection of excessive numbers of cycles with poor counts on certain projections.

Appearance
- Apparent perfusion defects can be created, the location of which depends on which projection(s) are affected.

Prevention
Either the acquisition can be repeated ungated, or gating parameters can be chosen to prevent loss of the more important perfusion data:
- Acquire each projection for a specific number of accepted cycles not for a fixed time: be aware that this may increase total acquisition time to an unacceptable duration.
- Increase the R-R acceptability window, to 100% if necessary: this may erode the reliability of gating indices.
- Acquire rejected cycles as a single extra 'frame' that can be added back into the summed static projections used to reconstruct perfusion slices.
- Some manufacturers' software allows simultaneous acquisition of both gated and ungated studies.

Recognition
- The raw data cine shows a heart that 'flashes' between projections, reflecting the varying counts.

Abnormal appearances in coronary artery disease

The aim of SPECT reporting is to identify abnormalities and differentiate them from normal variants. There is no substitute for an apprenticeship with an experienced reader in order to learn to appreciate common normal variants whilst recognizing sometimes subtle defects. Abnormal appearances should be described in the report according to extent and severity, and their clinical significance discussed.

A working knowledge of the following is an essential prerequisite to accurate reporting:

Coronary territories and their variation

- Right coronary artery.
- Left coronary artery.
- Coronary dominance.
- Coronary territories.

Perfusion defects

- Fixed defects.
- Reversible defects.
- Reverse redistribution.
- The problem of balanced multivessel disease.

Indirect markers of severe coronary artery disease

- Increased lung uptake of ^{201}Tl.
- Transient ischaemic dilatation (TID).
- Transient prominence of the right ventricular wall.
- Reversible impairment of LV function post stress.

Interpretation in LV dysfunction

- Exclusion of coronary disease in apparent dilated cardiomyopathy.
- Hibernating myocardium.

Appearances in non-coronary cardiac disease

- LBBB or ventricular pacing artefact.
- Dilated cardiomyopathy.
- Secondary LV hypertrophy.
- Hypertrophic cardiomyopathy (HCM).
- Congenital heart disease.

Coronary territories and their variation

The nuclear cardiologist requires a sound knowledge of the anatomy and territories of the coronary arteries to allow correlation with other clinical information, particularly when coronary angiography has already been performed.

Right coronary artery

- The right coronary artery (RCA) arises from the anterior aortic sinus and descends in the anterior atrioventricular groove, providing branches to the right atrium and right ventricle.
- At the crux (convergence of anterior and posterior atrioventricular, and inferior interventricular grooves), a dominant RCA divides into the posterior descending artery (PDA) and LV branch.
  - The PDA passes along the inferior interventricular groove towards the apex of the LV, supplying septal perforators to the inferior septum.
  - The LV branch courses distally in the posterior atrioventricular groove, giving off posterolateral branches to the inferolateral wall of the LV.

Left coronary artery

- The left coronary artery arises from the left posterior aortic sinus and, after a short course as the left mainstem behind the right ventricular outflow tract, divides into the left anterior descending (LAD) and cirumflex (LCx) arteries.
- The LAD runs in the anterior interventricular groove, all the way to the apex of the LV; it supplies:
  - Septal perforators to the anterior septum.
  - Diagonal branches to the anterolateral wall.
- The LCx runs behind the heart in the posterior atrioventricular groove, supplying obtuse marginal (OM) branches to the lateral wall; a distal non-dominant LCx tends to be small.

Coronary dominance

- In 85% of patients the RCA is said to be 'dominant', giving rise to the PDA and at least one posterolateral branch.
- In 7–8% the LCx is dominant, giving rise to the PDA and all of the posterolateral branches; the RCA is tiny.
- In the remaining 7–8% the RCA gives rise to the PDA and the LCx to all of the posterolateral branches (balanced or codominant circulation).

Coronary territories

There is marked variation in the myocardial territories of the coronary arteries between patients, particularly those of the RCA and LCx. As a rule, it is unwise to assign perfusion defects to specific coronary territories with too much confidence in the absence of angiographic information. Fig. 9.6 summarizes the segmental variations in coronary territories based on injection of a ^{99m}Tc-labelled perfusion tracer during angioplasty balloon inflation in patients with single-vessel coronary disease.

Some general rules are helpful:
- The territory of the LAD is usually the largest, accounting for approximately 50% of the LV myocardium.
- The anterior and anteroseptal walls are always supplied by the LAD.
- With the possible exception of the apical inferior segment, the apex is usually supplied by the LAD (unless there is a massive RCA or LCx with a vestigial LAD).
- The basal anterolateral wall is always supplied by the circumflex.
- The inferoseptal and apical inferior walls can be supplied by either the LAD or RCA, the inferior and inferolateral walls by either the RCA or LCx, and the mid anterolateral wall by either the LAD or LCx: the pattern of involvement of adjacent segments helps to distinguish between the possibilities.

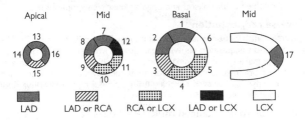

Fig. 9.6 Coronary territories and their variations according to the 17-segment model of the left ventricular myocardium, reproduced with permission.[1]

Reference

1 Pereztol-Valdés O, Candell-Riera J, Santana-Boado C, et al. Correspondence between left ventricular 17 myocardial segments and coronary arteries. Eur Heart J 2005; 26: 2637–43.

Perfusion defects

Fixed defects

A fixed defect exhibits no or minimal change in count density between stress and rest (Fig. 9.7). It suggests scar following previous infarction, or occasionally myocardial fibrosis as part of a non-coronary pathology. It should be described by location, extent and severity, using qualitative, semi-quantitative or quantitative techniques as required.

Reversible defects

A reversible defect shows improvement from stress to rest and suggests inducible hypoperfusion (Fig. 9.7). It should be described by location, extent, and severity, using qualitative, semi-quantitative or quantitative techniques as required. In practice, defects may be only partially reversible with a variable mixture of scar and ongoing inducible hypoperfusion.

Reverse redistribution

Reverse redistribution is a phenomenon mainly described with ^{201}Tl. The redistribution acquisition shows a paradoxical worsening of a perfusion defect compared with the initial stress study. This may reflect an area of non-transmural myocardial infarction subtended by a previously occluded but currently unobstructed coronary artery, producing increased washout of ^{201}Tl during redistribution.

The problem of balanced multivessel disease

Myocardial perfusion scintigraphy demonstrates *relative* myocardial perfusion, with the count density of each pixel within the myocardium colour-coded relative to the pixel of maximal counts. It follows that if all of the major epicardial coronary arteries were severely stenosed, producing global but uniform inducible hypoperfusion, then flow heterogeneity would not be readily detectable.

This is not simply a theoretical problem (see Fig. 9.8 on page 160). Whilst completely balanced hypoperfusion with entirely normal SPECT images is unusual, lesser degrees of the phenomenon may reduce the apparent extent and severity of perfusion defects, or mask all but the severest defects. Relatively minor defects may still be noted, but the severity of the underlying coronary disease may be underestimated. Important clues to the presence of more-or-less balanced multivessel disease include:

History
- High pre-test likelihood of disease:
  - Age.
  - Diabetes.
- Previously documented significant coronary disease.

Stress test
- Strongly positive exercise ECG.
- ST depression with vasodilator stress.

Indirect high-risk features on SPECT
- Increased lung uptake of ^{201}Tl.
- TID.
- Increased prominence of the right ventricular free wall with stress.
- Inducible regional or global LV dysfunction on post-stress gated acquisition.

(a)   (b)

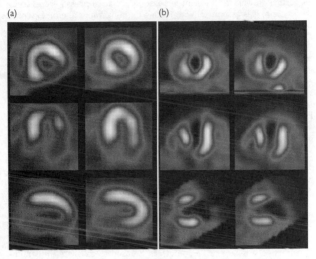

Fig. 9.7 Reversible inferolateral perfusion defect (a) and fixed apical perfusion defect (b). Left column stress, right column rest; top to bottom: short axis, horizontal long axis, vertical long axis. (See also colour plate section.)

Indirect markers of severe coronary artery disease

Increased lung uptake of ^{201}Tl

Exercise-induced increased lung uptake of ^{201}Tl (lung:heart ratio >0.8) suggests a chronic or transient increase in left atrial pressure due to LV dysfunction. It is associated with resting LV impairment and/or extensive coronary disease, and predicts a five- to six-fold increase in the risk of cardiac events.[1]

Transient ischaemic dilatation

Introduction

A dilated LV cavity on both stress and rest acquisitions suggests impaired systolic function at rest. In some patients with severe coronary disease, the cavity appears larger on the post-stress acquisition than at rest: TID. For optimal reporting confidence, TID should be visible on the raw data as well on the processed slices, and may be associated with a change to a more spherical shape of the LV.

Cause

TID is often said to reflect prolonged post-ischaemic stunning of LV function. However it may occur following vasodilator stress when true ischaemia is uncommon, and/or with ^{99m}Tc-labelled tracers when images are acquired 30–60 minutes post stress. An alternative explanation is that it represents diffuse subendocardial hypoperfusion with a false appearance of chamber dilatation.

Quantification

Quantitative software programmes can be used to calculate the volume within the LV endocardial border for both stress and rest slices, automatically generating a 'TID ratio' (stress volume/rest volume). A TID ratio of 1.2 is the upper limit of normal for an average sized LV.

Isolated TID

In the presence of perfusion defects, TID predicts severe coronary disease and a high risk of cardiac events. The interpretation of TID in the absence of a perfusion abnormality is more problematic (see Fig. 9.8). It may be the only clue to balanced multivessel coronary disease, but can also be a nonspecific finding, particularly in diabetes or LV hypertrophy. Isolated TID predicts a three- to four-fold increase in the risk of cardiac events, though given the low event rate (0.3% per year) following a fully normal study this still only equates to an absolute risk of cardiac death or nonfatal myocardial infarction of 1.1%.[2]

Transient prominence of the right ventricular wall

Ordinarily, the thin free wall of the right ventricle is hardly seen on SPECT. Transiently increased count density on the stress acquisition may occur if there is, in reality, global hypoperfusion of the LV myocardium.

Reversible impairment of LV function post stress

If both post-stress and rest acquisitions are gated, LV volumes and ejection fraction can be derived and compared. These global indices are reproducible, even for the low-dose part of a 1-day ^{99m}Tc protocol. A fall in ejection fraction of 5% or an increase in end-systolic volume of 10ml from rest to post-stress is significant, and may indicate severe ischaemia (equivalent to TID).

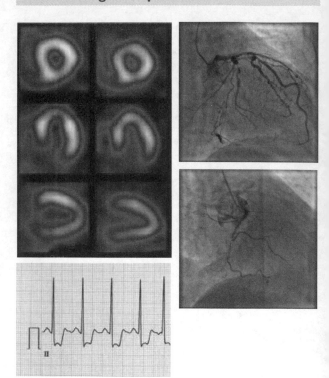

Fig. 9.8 Balanced multivessel coronary disease. A 76-year-old lady presented with a recent increase in her longstanding chest pain. SPECT slices (top left) demonstrated no definite perfusion defect, but there was (1) transient ischaemic dilatation of the left ventricular cavity with prominence of the right ventricular free wall; (2) a strongly positive exercise test, with limiting chest pain and deep ST depression at only 2 minutes 16 seconds of the modified Bruce protocol (bottom left). Subsequent coronary angiography demonstrated severe proximal three vessel coronary disease (right). (See also colour plate section.)

References

1 Gill JB, Ruddy TD, Newell JB, et al. Prognostic importance of thallium uptake by the lungs during exercise in coronary artery disease. *N Engl J Med* 1987; **317**: 1486–9.
2 Abidov A, Bax JJ, Hayes SW, et al. Transient ischemic dilation ratio of the left ventricle is a significant predictor of future cardiac events in patients with otherwise normal myocardial perfusion SPECT. *J Am Coll Cardiol* 2003; **42**: 1818–25.

Interpretation in LV dysfunction

MPS has two roles in patients with severe LV dysfunction but no angina:
- Exclusion of coronary disease as the underlying cause of an apparent dilated cardiomyopathy (see Fig. 9.9).
- Assessment of hibernating myocardium and the likely value of revascularization in patients with known coronary disease.

Exclusion of coronary disease in apparent dilated cardiomyopathy

A normal SPECT myocardial perfusion study excludes coronary disease in most cases: even patients with extensive hibernating myocardium usually have at least some scar.

Artefacts are common in dilated cardiomyopathy and should be recognized:
- LBBB with its characteristic artefact is often present.
- Inferior attenuation is exaggerated by LV dilatation.

Any definite perfusion abnormality, fixed as well as reversible, should usually prompt coronary angiography: inducible hypoperfusion may be underestimated or missed entirely in patients with multivessel disease.

Hibernating myocardium

Hibernating myocardium is:
- Dysfunctional at rest: demonstrable on gated SPECT.
- Viable (alive) as opposed to scar: takes up tracer at rest.
- Compromised by loss of vasodilator reserve, with hypoperfusion at rest or on minimal exertion: relatively reduced tracer uptake during stress.

Each of these features is readily assessed by routine SPECT myocardial perfusion scintigraphy. The presence of all three criteria is highly specific for functional improvement with revascularization. In one study, improvement with revascularization occurred in 80% of such segments, compared with only 30% of segments with viability and dysfunction but no reversibility.[1] Unfortunately inducible hypoperfusion is frequently underestimated, and so demonstration of the viability of dysfunctional segments is often considered sufficient, accepting a reduction in specificity as the price for adequate sensitivity.

Conventionally, myocardial segments whose count density is at least 50% of maximal counts are considered to contain sufficient viable myocardium to justify revascularization. Segments with count density 30–50% are likely to contain a mixture of viable myocardium and scar, but functional recovery is unlikely. A LV in which 25% or more of the myocardium remains viable is likely to improve with revascularization.

(a)   (b)

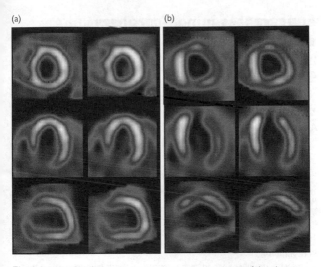

Fig. 9.9 Perfusion studies of two patients presenting with heart failure but no definite history of coronary disease or chest pain. (a) Dilated globular left ventricular cavity, with no perfusion abnormality; appearances typical of dilated cardiomyopathy. (b) Dilated left ventricular cavity, fixed apical perfusion defect, reversible lateral perfusion defect, possible inferior perfusion defect though attenuation likely; appearances strongly suggestive of ischaemic left ventricular dysfunction. Left column stress, right column rest; top short axis slice, middle horizontal long axis slice, bottom vertical long axis slice. (See also colour plate section.)

References

1 Kitsiou AN, Srinivasan G, Quyyumi AA, et al. Stress-induced reversible and mild-to-moderate irreversible thallium defects: are they equally accurate for predicting recovery of regional left ventricular function after revascularization? *Circulation* 1998; **98**: 501–8.

Appearances in non-coronary cardiac disease (1)

LBBB or ventricular pacing artefact

Cause
- Septal relaxation becomes increasingly dyssynchronous as heart rate increases, reducing septal perfusion relative to other walls.
- *Not* a problem with other conduction abnormalities.

Appearance
- Reversible septal perfusion defects are common in patients with LBBB or ventricular pacing stressed using exercise, in the absence of an explanatory coronary stenosis.
- LBBB may also produce fixed septal perfusion abnormalities, even when vasodilator stress is used.

Prevention
- Vasodilator stress with dipyridamole or adenosine (*not* combined with exercise) minimizes the problem as heart rate usually increases little; dobutamine should be avoided.

Recognition
- Defect is usually confined to the septum without involvement of the apex.

Dilated cardiomyopathy

Cause
- LBBB with its characteristic artefact is often present.
- Dilated LV cavity, with exaggeration of inferior attenuation.
- Patchy myocardial fibrosis can produce fixed defects.

Appearance
- Dilated LV cavity on both stress and rest acquisitions.
- Artefacts as above.

Recognition
- Typical appearance is a dilated LV with mildly reduced count density in the inferior wall and septum.
- Defects are usually not severe or reversible.
- Gated SPECT usually demonstrates global rather than regional hypokinesia.

There is no foolproof way of differentiating a myopathic process from extensive hibernating myocardium with severe underlying coronary disease, indeed patients with dilated cardiomyopathy may have real perfusion defects due to coincidental coronary disease. Coronary angiography should always be considered in equivocal cases.

Appearances in non-coronary cardiac disease (2)

Secondary LV hypertrophy

Cause
- Left ventricular hypertrophy can produce a variety of odd appearances in the absence of coronary disease.
- Apparent abnormalities are usually similar on stress and rest acquisitions.

Appearance
- Hypertrophy may produce generally increased count density throughout the LV myocardium, with sparing of the right ventricle.
- Localized papillary muscle hypertrophy can produce 'hot spots' in the inferior or lateral walls.

Recognition
- Clues are LV hypertrophy on the ECG, and vigorous contraction on gated SPECT.

Hypertrophic cardiomyopathy (HCM)

Cause
- Hypertrophic cardiomyopathy can produce a variety of appearances in the absence of coronary disease, depending on the location and degree of asymmetry of LV hypertrophy.

Appearance
- Predominant septal hypertrophy may produce a relative defect laterally.
- Apical hypertrophy can produce a 'hot spot' at the apex, with relatively reduced count density in the basal segments of the LV (Fig. 9.10).
- Reversibility may be seen in a grossly hypertrophied wall due to supply-demand imbalance, and is an adverse prognostic sign (Fig. 9.10).

Recognition
- ECG: LV hypertrophy with marked repolarization abnormalities.
- Echocardiogram: asymmetrical hypertrophy of the septum or apex, though may be concentric in some cases (NB apical HCM in particular can be missed on a suboptimal echo).
- Vigorous contraction on gated SPECT.

Congenital heart disease
- Prominent right ventricular free wall suggests hypertrophy due to pulmonary hypertension.
- Dextrocardia:
  - Should be apparent on cine of raw data if unsuspected: note position of liver.
  - Requires modification of orbit for acquisition: 180° from 45° left anterior oblique to 45° right posterior oblique, instead of the usual 45° right anterior oblique to 45° left posterior oblique.
  - Reconstructed and reorientated slices show inversion of septum and lateral wall.

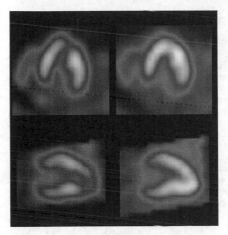

Fig. 9.10 Appearance in apical hypertrophic cardiomyopathy. Note the prominent apex on the rest acquisition, with an inducible apical perfusion abnormality during exercise. Left column stress, right column rest; top row horizontal long axis slice, bottom row vertical long axis slice. (See also colour plate section.)

Writing a useful report

Suggested structure

- **Patient details** and demographics.
- **Date** of study.
- **Heading**: for example, 'One-day exercise-rest tetrofosmin perfusion study with GTN at rest'.
- **Indication** for the study:
  - Previous cardiac history.
  - Results of other cardiac investigations, including previous myocardial perfusion scintigraphy or angiographic data if available.
  - Ongoing symptoms.
  - Specific clinical question.
- **Protocol**:
  - Tracer and protocol.
  - Doses injected.
  - Use of glyceryl trinitrate prior to resting injection.
- **Stress**:
  - Type and protocol: treadmill, bicycle, pharmacological.
  - Duration.
  - Symptoms and reason for stopping.
  - Haemodynamic response (heart rate and blood pressure).
  - Electrocardiogram at rest, during stress, and in recovery.
- **Findings**:
  - Quality issues from the raw data, mention motion correction if used.
  - Mention attenuation correction if used.
  - Non-cardiac abnormality if present.
  - Increased lung uptake of ^{201}Tl or dilatation of LV cavity if present.
  - For stress study, describe location, extent and severity of areas of reduced count density, from most to least severe.
  - For rest study, describe location, extent and completeness of any reversibility.
  - For gated acquisitions, describe location, extent and severity of wall motion abnormalities, comment on global LV function quoting volumes and ejection fraction, mention any improvement from post-stress to rest.
- **Conclusions**:
  - Comment on non-cardiac abnormality, increased lung uptake of ^{201}Tl, transient ischaemic dilatation, etc.
  - Confidently identify artefacts as such.
  - Summarize *real* perfusion defects in terms of location, extent, severity and degree of reversibility; unless angiographic data are available, it is usually wise to avoid assigning defects to specific coronary territories.
  - Describe LV function.
- A **'bottom line'** to the report is essential, cutting through the technical complexities for the referring clinician; depending on the clinical question, this might focus on one or more of the following:
  - Probability of obstructive coronary disease.
  - Origin of symptoms.

- Prognosis.
- Physiological relevance of documented angiographic stenoses.
- Value of angiography or revascularization.

Important points to remember

Review previous perfusion studies and coronary angiograms, if accessible.

Use a consistent and methodical approach to reporting, reviewing all available clinical, stress, and scintigraphic data. Always examine the looped cine of raw data for quality.

Calibrate the threshold for reporting abnormalities according to the clinical scenario. In general, a conservative approach is best: overenthusiastic reporting of minor apparent defects can lead to unnecessary normal coronary angiograms with a loss of confidence in the entire nuclear cardiology service, whilst missing the occasional true minor defect is unlikely to have major prognostic consequences. Conversely, in patients with proven coronary disease, an otherwise unconvincing abnormality may be harder to ignore: for example, a fixed defect consistent with anterior soft tissue attenuation in a woman with previous anterior myocardial infarction.

Avoid equivocation if at all possible. A statement such as 'possible inferior perfusion defect' in a patient who probably has inferior attenuation artefact is of little clinical value, and can easily lead to inappropriate coronary angiography. In cases where equivocation is genuinely unavoidable, the 'bottom-line' should consider the study overall and suggest an appropriate way forward (e.g. 'difficult to distinguish between fixed defect and artefact, but no reversibility and normal LV function so low risk study: conservative management appropriate').

Answer the clinical question, even when it is not fully articulated in the referral letter.

Liaise with the referring physician for difficult studies.

Remember that myocardial perfusion scintigraphy is a physiological technique whilst coronary angiography is anatomical. Do not be demoralized when the results of the two investigations appear discordant: it does not necessarily follow that the functional test is 'wrong'.

Chapter 10

Myocardial perfusion scintigraphy: clinical value

Diagnosis and exclusion of coronary artery disease (1)

Myocardial perfusion scintigraphy (MPS) is most commonly used to diagnose or exclude obstructive coronary disease in patients presenting with chest pain. A Bayesian approach is traditionally used, taking coronary angiography as the 'gold standard'. A clinical pre-test likelihood of disease is estimated based on age, sex, and history (see Tables 10.1 and 10.2). This is subsequently refined into a post-test likelihood utilizing the result of a diagnostic test of known sensitivity (proportion of positive tests in patients with coronary disease) and specificity (proportion of negative test in patients without coronary disease).

If the test is positive:

$$\text{Post-test odds} = \text{pre-test odds} \times \frac{\text{sensitivity}}{1 - \text{specificity}}$$

If the test is negative:

$$\text{Post-test odds} = \text{pre-test odds} \times \frac{1 - \text{sensitivity}}{\text{specificity}}$$

Note:

$$\text{'odds'} = \frac{\text{probability}}{1 - \text{probability}}$$

This gives rise to curves such as those in Fig. 10.1, which illustrate that any test has its greatest discriminatory value in patients at intermediate risk of disease.

Limitations of the exercise electrocardiogram

The exercise electrocardiogram (ECG) is the most available and easiest test to perform in patients with chest pain. Its use is supported by a large body of evidence, and its sensitivity and specificity are typically 70% in the literature.[1]

The exercise ECG performs particularly poorly in some important groups of patient:
• Patients unable to exercise maximally due to arthritis, lung disease, etc.
• Women, who typically exercise to lower workload than men and in whom false positive ST depression is frequent.
• Patients with important resting ECG abnormalities, particularly left bundle branch block or ventricular pacing.

- Patients with significant hypertension, where elevated blood pressure forces early termination or repolarization abnormalities are present on the resting ECG.
- Diabetics, who are often unable to exercise maximally.
- Patients in atrial fibrillation, where exercise capacity may be poor due to abruptly increasing heart rate, or digoxin therapy may produce false positive ST depression.
- Asian and African patients, who have a higher rate of inconclusive results.

Moreover, patients are being investigated with lower and lower pre-test likelihoods of coronary disease (e.g. as part of health screening), in whom the exercise ECG is of poor discriminatory value.

Table 10.1 Evaluation of chest pain[2]

Score	Symptoms described
Typical (definite) angina	Substernal chest pain of characteristic quality and duration
	Provoked by exertion or emotional stress
	Relieved by rest or GTN
Atypical (probable) angina	2 out of 3 above symptoms
Non-cardiac pain	1 or none of the above symptoms

(GTN = glyceryl trinitrate)

Table 10.2 Probability (%) of angiographic coronary disease according to age, sex, and symptoms[3]

Age	Non-cardiac chest pain		Atypical angina		Typical angina	
	Male	Female	Male	Female	Male	Female
30–39	5	1	22	4	70	26
40–49	14	3	46	13	87	55
50–59	22	8	59	32	92	79
60–69	28	19	67	54	94	91

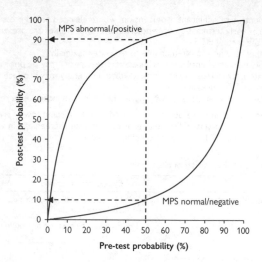

Fig. 10.1 Bayesian approach to diagnosis of coronary disease using MPS, assuming sensitivity 90% and specificity 90%.[4] The difference in post-test probability between abnormal (positive) and normal (negative) MPS is maximal at intermediate pre-test probability.

References

1 Detrano R, Gianrossi R, Froelicher V. The diagnostic accuracy of the exercise electrocardiogram: a meta-analysis of 22 years of research. *Prog Cardiovasc Dis* 1989; **32**: 173–206.

2 Diamond GA. A clinically relevant classification of chest discomfort. *J Am Coll Cardiol* 1983; **1**: 574–5.

3 Diamond GA, Forrester JS. Analysis of probability as an aid in the clinical diagnosis of coronary artery disease. *N Engl J Med* 1979; **300**: 1350–8.

4 Loong CY, Anagnostopoulos C. Diagnosis of coronary artery disease by radionuclide myocardial perfusion imaging. *Heart* 2004; **90**(Suppl5): v2–9.

Diagnosis and exclusion of coronary artery disease (2)

Value of MPS

The diagnostic value of MPS is firmly established for every combination of stress technique and tracer protocol. Planar imaging remains valuable in some situations, but has been largely superseded by single photon emission computed tomography (SPECT) which offers superior diagnostic sensitivity, particularly when only single vessel coronary disease is present. The sensitivity of SPECT across a large number of studies is approximately 90%.[1] The calculated specificity is typically lower, and has varied greatly between studies. The best studies have achieved specificities of approximately 75%, which increases when gated data are included.

Problems with published values of sensitivity and specificity

The true specificity of MPS has probably been underestimated in many studies for two reasons:

- The ability of experienced reporters to 'read around a defect' was not applied, with obvious artefacts being erroneously classified as perfusion defects.
- Post-test referral bias means that patients with abnormal perfusion scintigraphy are more likely to undergo 'gold standard' coronary angiography than those with normal imaging; this leads to identification of almost all 'false positive' tests, whilst underestimating the number of 'true negative' tests.

In practice, a more meaningful alternative to specificity is the normalcy rate, defined as the proportion of normal tests in a population with a low probability (<5%) of coronary disease based on clinical factors. Normalcy rates for MPS are typically 90% or more.

Values for the overall sensitivity of MPS obscure the fact that the test is better at identifying multivessel coronary disease than single vessel disease (sensitivity as low as 80%). For single vessel disease, sensitivity for stenoses in the left anterior descending artery is higher than that for stenoses in the right coronary or circumflex arteries, probably reflecting its larger territory.

Problems with the Bayesian approach

The Bayesian approach to the investigation of suspected coronary disease originated in an era when coronary angiography was the only means of imaging the coronary circulation, and revascularization with bypass surgery the only effective treatment. Today the situation is more complex: coronary angiography remains the 'gold standard' for coronary luminal stenoses and guiding revascularization, but other investigations are available which can define other aspects of coronary pathophysiology, and effective pharmacological treatments are available which can improve both prognosis and symptoms.

An uncritical Bayesian approach to the use of MPS is therefore unhelpful. MPS, a functional test, and coronary angiography, an anatomical test, reveal entirely different but valid aspects of coronary disease, and it should not be surprising that the two investigations yield apparently contradictory results in some patients. For example, a normal MPS study in a patient subsequently found to have coronary stenoses at angiography might be dismissed as a 'false positive'. However, in more sophisticated hands, the same normal MPS study performed *after* angiography in exactly the same patient would provide valuable reassurance from a prognostic and symptomatic point of view.

References

1 Underwood SR, Anagnostopoulos C, Cerqueira M, *et al.* Myocardial perfusion scintigraphy: The evidence. *Eur J Nucl Med Mol Imaging* 2004; **31**: 261–91.

Cost-effectiveness in diagnosis of coronary artery disease

MPS is clinically effective in the diagnosis of coronary artery disease. However, it is a more expensive investigation than the exercise ECG, whilst being less accurate (by definition) than coronary angiography. On the other hand, MPS has a diagnostic accuracy which is superior to the exercise ECG, and might help to avoid a proportion of more expensive normal angiograms. In the planning of cardiac services, it is important to know whether diagnostic strategies which employ MPS are cost-effective compared with alternatives which do not.

MPS compared with direct coronary angiography

The Economics of Noninvasive Diagnosis (END) Study was an American study which retrospectively compared 5423 patients investigated directly by coronary angiography with 5826 patients investigated by MPS as a first-line test.[1] 34% of the MPS patients subsequently underwent angiography. The rates of cardiac events over 3 years were comparable between the two strategies at every level of pre-test clinical risk. However, the cost of care per patient over the same period was 30–40% lower for those undergoing MPS as the first-line investigation.

MPS compared with exercise ECG

In the Economics of Myocardial Perfusion Imaging in Europe (EMPIRE) Study, there was no difference in outcome over 2 years between a strategy which relied on the exercise ECG alone followed by angiography as appropriate (146 patients), compared with one which employed the exercise ECG followed by MPS followed by angiography as appropriate (131 patients).[2] However, the management cost per patient over the same period was lower using the MPS strategy by 14% for those with coronary disease and by 33% for those without coronary disease.

The EMPIRE Study was conducted retrospectively, but a more recent study randomized 457 outpatients with chest pain to first-line exercise ECG or MPS.[3] Compared with exercise ECG, MPS reduced the proportion of patients at intermediate post-test probability of disease (that is, effectively undiagnosed) from 30% to 3%, and the proportion undergoing coronary angiography from 47% to 16%. In patients at low pre-test probability of disease, a strategy of first-line MPS was more expensive than exercise ECG. For patients at intermediate or high pre-test probability, depending on the exact costs used in calculation, first-line MPS was either no more expensive than exercise ECG or significantly cheaper.

Conclusion

The use of MPS in the investigation of chest pain is more cost-effective than direct coronary angiography. The literature does not support the use of MPS as an alternative to first-line exercise ECG in all patients. Nevertheless, it is likely that the selective use of MPS in patients who have, or are likely to have, an equivocal exercise ECG *is* cost-effective, in addition to avoiding unnecessary invasive investigation.

References

1 Shaw LJ, Hachamovitch R, Berman DS, et al. The economic consequences of available diagnostic and prognostic strategies for the evaluation of stable angina patients: An observational assessment of the value of precatheterization ischemia. *J Am Coll Cardiol* 1999; **33**: 661–9.

2 Underwood SR, Godman B, Salyani S, et al. Economics of myocardial perfusion imaging in Europe – the EMPIRE study. *Eur Heart J* 1999; **20**: 157–66.

3 Sabharwal NK, Stoykova B, Taneja AK, et al. A randomized trial of exercise treadmill ECG versus stress SPECT myocardial perfusion imaging as an initial diagnostic strategy in stable patients with chest pain and suspected CAD: Cost analysis. *J Nucl Cardiol* 2007; **14**: 174–86.

Prognosis in suspected stable coronary artery disease

MPS provides robust prognostic as well as diagnostic data in stable patients with suspected coronary disease. Several studies involving thousands of patients have been sufficiently large to allow the predictive value of various MPS parameters to be defined for individual cardiac end-points. In general, the more abnormal a MPS study is overall, the worse the prognosis.

Prognostic value of a normal study

The major cardiac event rate (cardiac death or non-fatal myocardial infarction) following a normal MPS study has been studied for every combination of stress technique and tracer protocol and is consistently less than 1% per year. A meta-analysis of 14 studies published between 1994 and 1997, involving more than 12 000 patients followed for a mean of 20 months, yielded an annual event rate of 0.6%.[1] Patients with chest pain but a normal MPS study therefore have a prognosis which is comparable with the asymptomatic population. Coronary angiography is seldom indicated in such patients.

Importantly, the annual event rate remains low following a normal MPS study for approximately 5 years, before returning to that of the population to which the patient belongs.[2] This gives rise to the concept of a 'warranty period' after a normal study, during which repeat MPS testing is unlikely to be indicated.

Prognostic value of an abnormal study

Patients with an abnormal MPS study are at increased risk of cardiac events, though the exact rate depends on the population and degree to which the study is abnormal. In their meta-analysis, Iskander and Iskandrian demonstrated a major cardiac event rate of 7.4% per year overall.[1]

MPS has incremental prognostic value over other clinical and exercise electrocardiographic indices, including the Duke treadmill score.[3] However it is worth remembering that the converse is also true and that these other sources of information should be used to refine a MPS-based assessment of risk.

Increasingly abnormal MPS studies confer an increasingly worse prognosis. In particular, increasingly extensive inducible hypoperfusion leads to an increasing rate of non-fatal myocardial infarction, whilst worsening left ventricular function on gated SPECT leads to an increasing rate of cardiac death (Fig. 10.2).[4] Other adverse MPS features, such as increased lung uptake of ^{201}Tl or transient ischaemic dilatation of the left ventricular cavity, further increase the cardiac event rate for a given extent of perfusion abnormality. Interestingly, the presence of marked transient ischaemic dilatation in a patient with an otherwise normal MPS study increases the annual event rate to nearly 2%.[5]

Concept of 'modifiable' risk

The identification of patients at high risk of cardiac events is of little practical value unless that risk can be reduced by medical intervention. Retrospective data from Cedars-Sinai indicate that the extent of reversible hypoperfusion on MPS predicts not only the absolute risk of cardiac events, but also the relative prognostic benefit of coronary revascularization over medical management (the 'modifiable' component of risk: see Fig. 10.3).[6] Unless 10% or more of the myocardium is ischaemic on a MPS study, revascularization does not confer prognostic benefit over conservative management and coronary angiography cannot easily be justified on prognostic grounds (though there might be a symptomatic indication).

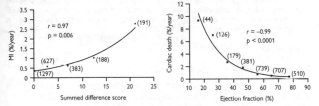

Fig. 10.2 Risk of non-fatal myocardial infarction and cardiac death as separate functions of the extent of inducible hypoperfusion (summed difference score) and left ventricular ejection fraction (2686 patients followed for mean 21 months), reproduced with permission.[1]

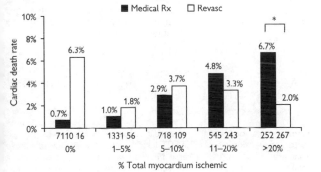

Fig. 10.3 Annual cardiac death rate according to the percentage of myocardium with inducible hypoperfusion, stratified by management (10 627 patients followed for mean 2 years), reproduced with permission.[6]

References

1 Iskander S, Iskandrian AE. Risk assessment using single-photon emission computed tomographic technetium-99m sestamibi imaging. *J Am Coll Cardiol* 1998; **32**: 57–62.

2 Hachamovitch R, Hayes S, Friedman JD, *et al.* Determinants of risk and its temporal variation in patients with normal stress myocardial perfusion scans. *J Am Coll Cardiol* 2003; **41**: 1329–40.

3 Hachamovitch R, Berman DS, Kiat H, *et al.* Exercise myocardial perfusion SPECT in patients without known coronary artery disease: incremental prognostic value and use in risk stratification. *Circulation* 1996; **93**: 905–14.

4 Sharir T, Germano G, Kang X, *et al.* Prediction of myocardial infarction versus cardiac death by gated myocardial perfusion SPECT: risk stratification by the amount of stress-induced ischemia and the poststress ejection fraction. *J Nucl Med* 2001; **42**: 831–7.

5 Abidov A, Bax JJ, Hayes SW, *et al.* Transient ischemic dilatation ratio of the left ventricle is a significant predictor of future cardiac events in patients with otherwise normal myocardial perfusion SPECT. *J Am Coll Cardiol* 2003; **42**: 1818–25.

6 Hachamovitch R, Hayes SW, Friedman JD, *et al.* Comparison of the short-term survival benefit associated with revascularization compared with medical therapy in patients with no prior coronary artery disease undergoing stress myocardial perfusion single photon emission computed tomography. *Circulation* 2003; **107**: 2900–6.

Risk assessment prior to elective non-cardiac surgery

Technological advances in surgical techniques and perioperative care have greatly reduced the cardiac risk of non-cardiac surgery. However, in an era when postoperative outcomes are the subject of intense scrutiny, there is an increasing need to identify high-risk patients prior to surgery. MPS is frequently used to assess the perioperative coronary risk of stable patients prior to elective non-cardiac surgery, but should be used selectively and only as part of a carefully considered management strategy.

General approach

Consider nature and urgency of surgery

- Urgent life-saving surgery should not be delayed due to misplaced concerns about cardiac risk.
- Certain types of surgery (e.g. peripheral vascular procedures) carry an inherently high cardiac risk.

Consider patient's clinical status

- Patients with ongoing symptoms of coronary disease (i.e. angina) should generally undergo cardiological assessment irrespective of the need for non-cardiac surgery.
- Consider using a simple scoring system to quantify clinical risk (see Tables 10.3 and 10.4).[1,2]

Assess indication for specialized testing, such as MPS

- Focus on patients in whom clinical assessment alone gives insufficient reassurance (i.e. those at intermediate risk).
- Exercise ECG is a reasonable first-line test, reserving MPS or stress echo for those unsuitable.
- Left ventricular systolic function, whether assessed using radionuclide ventriculography, echocardiography, or gated SPECT, is a poor predictor of perioperative risk (which is largely determined by the risk of acute ischaemic events), though a good predictor of longer-term risk.

Value of MPS prior to non-cardiac surgery

- Absence of inducible hypoperfusion predicts low risk of postoperative cardiac death or non-fatal myocardial infarction (e.g. 1–2% post vascular surgery).
- Presence of inducible hypoperfusion more difficult to interpret, for example, in vascular patients:
  - Common finding (25–50%).
  - Risk of postoperative cardiac event still 'only' 10–25%.
  - Risk increases with extent of abnormality, but remains <50% for even the most ischaemic studies.

Cardiological management post MPS

Patients with mild or moderate ischaemia on functional testing should be carefully β-blocked perioperatively.[3] Coronary angiography should usually be reserved for patients who require the investigation independently of the proposed non-cardiac surgery (e.g. for angina), as revascularization purely to lower perioperative risk is generally ineffective.[4] The exception may be patients with very extensive ischaemia (>25% of left ventricular myocardium) who cannot be adequately protected by β-blockade.[5] However recent data suggest that even these are not helped by revascularization.[6]

Table 10.3 Revised Cardiac Risk Index for clinical assessment prior to general surgery[1]

Risk factor	Definition
High-risk surgery	AAA repair, thoracic, abdominal
Ischaemic heart disease	MI, Q-waves, nitrates, +ve exercise test
Congestive heart failure	history, examination, chest radiograph
Cerebrovascular disease	stroke, transient ischaemic attack
Insulin-treated diabetes	
Renal dysfunction	creatinine >177μmol/l

Number of factors	Proportion of patients	Cardiac events
0	36%	0.4%
1	39%	1.1%
2	18%	4.6%
3	7%	9.7%

Table 10.4 Eagle Score for clinical assessment prior to peripheral vascular surgery[2]

Risk factor	
Age ≥70	Myocardial infarction (history or Q-waves)
Diabetes	Congestive heart failure
Angina	

Number of factors	Proportion	LMS or 3v disease	Cardiac events
0	30–40%	5%	3%
1–2	50%	16%	8%
≥3	10–20%	43%	18%

(LMS = left mainstem, 3v = three-vessel)

References

1 Lee TH, Marcantonio ER, Mangione CM, *et al.* Derivation and prospective validation of a simple index for prediction of cardiac risk of major noncardiac surgery. *Circulation* 1999; **100**: 1043–9.

2 L'Italien GJ, Paul SD, Hendel RC, *et al.* Development and validation of a Bayesian model for perioperative cardiac risk assessment in a cohort of 1,081 vascular surgical candidates. *J Am Coll Cardiol* 1996; **27**: 779–86.

3 Poldermans D, Boersma E, Bax JJ, *et al.* The effect of bisoprolol on perioperative mortality and myocardial infarction in high-risk patients undergoing vascular surgery. *N Engl J Med* 1999; **341**: 1789–94.

4 McFalls EO, Ward HB, Moritz TE, *et al.* Coronary-artery revascularization before elective major vascular surgery. *N Engl J Med* 2004; **351**: 2795–804.

5 Boersma E, Poldermans D, Bax JJ, *et al.* Predictors of cardiac events after major vascular surgery: role of clinical characteristics, dobutamine echocardiography, and beta-blocker therapy. *JAMA* 2001; **285**: 1865–73.

6 Poldermans D, Schouten O, Vidakovic R, *et al.* A clinical randomized trial to evaluate the safety of a noninvasive approach to high-risk patients undergoing major vascular surgery. The DECREASE-V Pilot Study. *J Am Coll Cardiol* 2007; **49**: 1763–9.

Special groups: women

The assessment of coronary disease in women presents particular challenges compared with men:
- Clinicians may exercise an inadequate level of suspicion.
- Symptoms may be atypical.
- Risk particularly high for those with diabetes.
- Exercise ECG performs poorly:
  - Lower pre-test probability.
  - Lower exercise capacity.
  - ST depression less specific.
- Smaller evidence base because of under-representation in clinical studies.

Diagnosis of coronary disease

MPS is consistently better than the exercise ECG in the diagnosis or exclusion of coronary disease in women. A review of seven studies including 1140 women reported a mean sensitivity of 78% and specificity 86%.[1]

Anterior attenuation artefact is a particular problem in women, and would be expected to erode the specificity of MPS. This has been a decreasing problem with progressive technical advances such as the introduction of Tc-labelled tracers and gated SPECT (Fig. 10.4).[2]

Prognosis

The prognostic value of MPS in women is at least as good as that in men. In one large study (2742 men, 1394 women), the cardiac event rate following a normal MPS study was similarly low in men and women, but following an abnormal study was highest in women (see Fig. 10.5).[3] Moreover, the incremental prognostic value of MPS over clinical and exercise variables was greatest in women (Fig. 10.6).

Cost-effectiveness

The use of MPS in women as a gatekeeper to coronary angiography is cost-effective across the spectrum of pre-test probabilities.[4]

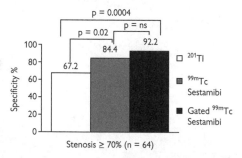

Fig. 10.4 Specificity of MPS in women using ^{201}Tl, ^{99m}Tc-sestamibi, and gating, reproduced with permission.[2]

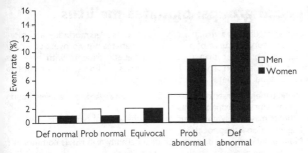

Fig. 10.5 Cardiac event rate in men and women according to degree of abnormality of MPS study, reproduced with permission.[3]

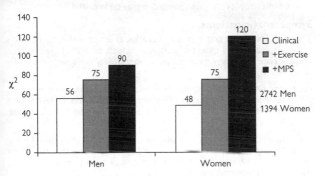

Fig. 10.6 Incremental prognostic value of MPS in men and women, reproduced with permission.[3]

References

1 Iskandrian AE, Heo J, Nallamothu N. Detection of coronary artery disease in women with use of stress single-photon emission computed tomography myocardial perfusion imaging. *J Nucl Cardiol* 1997; **4**: 329–35.

2 Taillefer R, DePuey EG, Udelson JE, et al. Comparative diagnostic accuracy of Tl-201 and Tc 99m sestamibi SPECT imaging (perfusion and ECG-gated SPECT) in detecting coronary artery disease in women. *J Am Coll Cardiol* 1997; **29**: 69–77.

3 Hachamovitch R, Berman DS, Kiat H, et al. Effective risk stratification using exercise myocardial perfusion SPECT in women: gender-related differences in prognostic nuclear testing. *J Am Coll Cardiol* 1996; **28**: 34–44.

4 Shaw LJ, Heller GV, Travin MI, et al. Cost analysis of diagnostic testing for coronary artery disease in women with stable chest pain. *J Nucl Cardiol* 1999; **6**: 559–69.

Special groups: diabetes mellitus

Diabetes mellitus is a major cause of cardiovascular morbidity and mortality. The survival curve of patients with diabetes but no overt coronary disease is no better than that of non-diabetic patients with previous myocardial infarction. This has led the various cardiovascular societies to consider type 2 diabetes as a 'coronary equivalent'.

Diabetic patients present certain challenges with regard to the investigation and treatment of coronary disease:
- Patients may be asymptomatic or describe atypical symptoms (e.g. exertional dyspnoea).
- Multivessel coronary disease with its inherently high risk is common.
- Exercise electrocardiography performs poorly:
  - Exercise capacity may be impaired due to obesity, peripheral vascular disease, etc.
  - Chronotropic response to exercise may be impaired.

Symptomatic patients

The rate of major cardiac events in diabetics, as in non-diabetics, increases with the severity and extent of perfusion defects on MPS. However, the risk associated with any given perfusion abnormality is higher, particularly in women (Fig. 10.7).[1]

Even after a normal MPS study the cardiac risk appears to be higher in diabetics than in non-diabetics. This is best understood in terms of a reduction in the 'warranty period' from 5 years down to 2 years or less, particularly in women.[2]

For a given MPS result, type 1 diabetics are at higher risk than type 2 diabetics. Similarly, those presenting with dyspnoea are at substantially higher risk than those presenting with angina, who in turn are at higher risk than asymptomatic patients (Fig. 10.8).[3]

Asymptomatic patients

The concept of using MPS to screen asymptomatic diabetics for significant coronary disease is being increasingly discussed, even though there is little evidence that revascularizing such patients is of prognostic value. The Detection of Ischaemia in Asymptomatic Diabetics (DIAD) study examined the prevalence of abnormal MPS in 522 diabetics in the community.[4] Silent ischaemia was identified in 22%, but only 0.8% had a perfusion defect amounting to ≥10% of the left ventricular myocardium: that is, more than 1000 patients would have to be screened to find one whose prognosis might be improved by revascularization. Thus MPS as a primary screening tool is unlikely to be cost-effective, though it might have merit as a second-line test for patients with, for example, a high computed tomography (CT) coronary calcification score.[5]

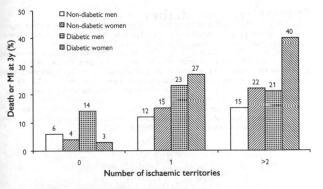

Fig. 10.7 Annual cardiac event rate as a function of the extent of ischaemia in non-diabetic and diabetic men and women, reproduced with permission.[1]

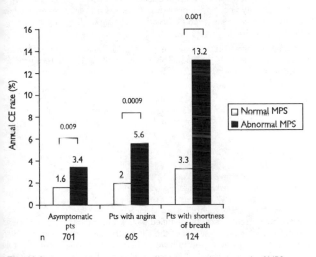

Fig. 10.8 Annual cardiac event rate in diabetics according to result of MPS and presenting symptom, reproduced with permission.[3]

References

1 Giri S, Shaw LJ, Murthy DR, *et al.* Impact of diabetes on the risk stratification using stress single-photon emission computed tomography myocardial perfusion imaging in patients with symptoms suggestive of coronary artery disease. *Circulation* 2002; **105**: 32–40.

2 Hachamovitch R, Hayes S, Friedman JD, *et al.* Determinants of risk and its temporal variation in patients with normal stress myocardial perfusion scans. *J Am Coll Cardiol* 2003; **41**: 1329–40.

3 Zellweger MJ, Hachamovitch R, Kang X, *et al.* Prognostic relevance of symptoms versus objective evidence of coronary artery disease in diabetic patients. *Eur Heart J* 2004; **25**: 543–50.

4 Wackers FJT, Young LH, Inzucchi SE, *et al.* Detection of silent myocardial ischemia in asymptomatic diabetic subjects. *Diabetes Care* 2004; **27**: 1954–61.

5 Anand DV, Lim E, Hopkins D, *et al.* Risk stratification in uncomplicated type 2 diabetes: prospective evaluaton of the combined use of coronary artery calcium imaging and selective myocardial perfusion scintigraphy. *Eur Heart J* 2006; **27**: 713–21.

Assessment in known stable coronary artery disease

The prognostic value of MPS extends even to patients already proven to have coronary disease. Indeed, even angiographic data add nothing to a proportional hazards model which already contains MPS data.[1]

As in patients without proven coronary disease, a normal MPS study in patients with documented disease confers a low risk of cardiac events, though the 'warranty period' is considerably shorter: for example, for a 60-year-old non-diabetic male the annual risk remains below 1% for 7 years in the absence of proven coronary disease, but for as little as 1 year in its presence.[2]

After coronary angiography

MPS may be valuable after coronary angiography to assess the functional significance of anatomical stenoses and hence the need for revascularization.

From a prognostic point of view, only patients with inducible hypoperfusion affecting at least 10% of the left ventricular myocardium are likely to derive prognostic benefit from revascularization; below this threshold, medical management is associated with a lower cardiac event rate (see Fig. 10.3 on page 181).[3]

From a symptomatic point of view, MPS can be used to uncover the origin of atypical symptoms in patients with proven angiographic stenoses, or identify which of several possible targets for revascularization is/are the most flow-limiting. In this context it should be noted that the pattern of ST depression on an exercise ECG provides no localizing information.

After revascularization

Following coronary artery bypass graft surgery (CABG), MPS provides prognostic data whether performed early (<2 years) or late (>5 years), even in asymptomatic individuals.[4]

Following percutaneous coronary intervention (PCI), a normal MPS study in a patient with an early recurrence of chest pain is reassuring. However, inducible perfusion defects due to residual microvascular dysfunction are common within 2 months of successful PCI, and in general patients may be better served by repeat angiography. Later after PCI, MPS is of clearer clinical value.

References

1 Iskandrian AS, Chae SC, Heo J, et al. Independent and incremental prognostic value of exercise single-photon emission computed tomographic (SPECT) thallium imaging in coronary artery disease. *J Am Coll Cardiol* 1993; **22**: 665–70.

2 Hachamovitch R, Hayes S, Friedman JD, et al. Determinants of risk and its temporal variation in patients with normal stress myocardial perfusion scans. *J Am Coll Cardiol* 2003; **41**: 1329–40.

3 Hachamovitch R, Hayes SW, Friedman JD, et al. Comparison of the short-term survival benefit associated with revascularization compared with medical therapy in patients with no prior coronary artery disease undergoing stress myocardial perfusion single photon emission computed tomography. *Circulation* 2003; **107**: 2900–6.

4 Lauer MS, Lytle B, Pashkow F, et al. Prediction of death and myocardial infarction by screening with exercise-thallium testing after coronary-artery-bypass grafting. *Lancet* 1998; **351**: 615–22.

Assessment following proven acute coronary syndrome

The assessment, classification and management of acute coronary syndromes has become increasingly complex over the last 20 years, and the role of MPS has evolved accordingly.

ST-elevation myocardial infarction (STEMI)

Acute phase

Patients presenting with STEMI require immediate coronary reperfusion, whether by thrombolysis or primary angioplasty, and MPS has no decision-making role in the acute phase. It may nevertheless be a useful research tool, as injection of a ^{99m}Tc-labelled perfusion tracer prior to reperfusion continues to define the ischaemic area at risk on a scan acquired a few hours later, whilst a further injection a week or so later defines the final infarct size. The difference between the two perfusion defects reflects the amount of myocardial salvage, and this has been a useful end-point in a number of studies of adjuvant therapies in reperfusion.

Recovery phase

Once a patient has stabilized, MPS becomes a valuable clinical tool in risk stratification, with its ability to define both ischaemic burden and left ventricular function (on gated SPECT). Vasodilator stress can be used safely as early as day 2 post-infarct as it provokes coronary hyperaemia without increasing myocardial oxygen demand. The multicentre adenosine sestamibi SPECT post-infarction evaluation (INSPIRE) study demonstrated that adenosine ^{99m}Tc-sestamibi SPECT used in this way predicted cardiac events at one year independently of Thrombolysis In Myocardial Infarction (TIMI) Risk Score and left ventricular ejection fraction (Table 10.5).[1] This was despite the fact that revascularization rates increased across the risk groups. Low-risk patients were discharged earlier from hospital and derived no prognostic benefit from revascularization.

Non-STEMI and unstable angina pectoris (NSTEMI/UAP)

The management of NSTEMI/UAP has evolved rapidly. Earlier controversy about whether early intervention is generally superior to medical therapy has given way to arguments about *which* patients stand to benefit.

Patients with high risk clinical features such as elevated troponins or ST depression benefit from early intervention. Lower risk patients are better candidates for non-invasive risk assessment with MPS. In a meta-analysis, the absence of inducible hypoperfusion predicted a low risk (2%), whereas its presence predicted high risk (24%); in contrast, exercise ECG data were poorly discriminatory.[2]

Table 10.5 Outcome of 728 stable survivors of myocardial infarction, stratified by results of early adenosine ^{99m}Tc-sestamibi SPECT.[1] CD/MI = cardiac death or non-fatal myocardial infarction.

Perfusion defect	Patients	Revascularized	Inpatient stay (days)	1y CD/MI
Stress <20%	33%	16%	5.5	1.8%
Stress ≥20% Reversible <10%	29%	21%	8.0	9.2%
Stress ≥20% Reversible ≥10%	38%	64%	13.9	11.6%

References

1 Mahmarian JJ, Shaw LJ, Filipchuk NG, et al. A multinational study to establish the value of early adenosine technetium-99m sestamibi myocardial perfusion imaging in identifying a low-risk group for early hospital discharge after acute myocardial infarction. *J Am Coll Cardiol* 2006; **48**: 2448–57.

2 Brown KA. Management of unstable angina: the role of noninvasive risk stratification. *J Nucl Cardiol* 1997; **4**: S164–8.

Assessment of acute chest pain

Acute chest pain is a common reason for attendance at the Emergency Department. Patients with a non-diagnostic ECG commonly undergo serial troponin measurements, followed by risk assessment with exercise electrocardiography or coronary angiography as appropriate. Overnight admissions are frequent and expensive.

Early resting SPECT imaging has similar sensitivity to serial troponins over 24 hours, but is far superior to initial troponin alone. It therefore offers earlier exclusion of an acute coronary syndrome, potentially avoiding unnecessary admission.

Practical considerations

^{99m}Tc-labelled tracers are more convenient than ^{201}Tl as.
• Available 24 hours a day from the hospital radiopharmacy.
• Imaging can be delayed for logistical reasons without redistribution.

The dose of radiopharmaceutical is injected as soon as possible after presentation. Perfusion defects are detectable for several hours following the resolution of chest pain, though diagnostic sensitivity declines after 4 hours.

Patients with normal resting MPS can be safely discharged, but are usually brought back for an outpatient stress study to complete the assessment. Patients with abnormal resting MPS require admission for aggressive treatment.

Clinical value

A number of studies have demonstrated a very high (>99%) negative predictive value for excluding an acute coronary syndrome.[1] More importantly, patients with normal MPS are at very low risk: the rate of myocardial infarction at 30 days is <1% with a normal study versus 10% with an abnormal study.[2]

The Emergency Room Assessment of Sestamibi for Evaluation (ERASE) Chest Pain Trial demonstrated the value of MPS in 'real-life' decision-making. 2475 patients with chest pain and a non-diagnostic ECG were randomized to acute ^{99m}Tc-sestamibi SPECT versus routine management. Outcome at 30 days was similar between the groups. Whilst triage decisions were comparable for patients *with* an acute coronary syndrome, the admission rate was reduced from 52 to 42% for those *without* an acute coronary syndrome.[2]

1 Heller GV, Stowers SA, Hendel RC, et al. Clinical value of acute rest technetium-99m tetrofosmin tomographic myocardial perfusion imaging in patients with acute chest pain and nondiagnostic electrocardiograms. J Am Coll Cardiol 1998; **31**: 1011–7.
2 Udelson JE, Beshansky JR, Ballin DS, et al. Myocardial perfusion imaging for evaluation and triage of patients with suspected acute cardiac ischemia: a randomized controlled trial. JAMA 2002; **288**: 2693–700.

Assessment for hibernating myocardium (1)

In patients with ischaemic left ventricular dysfunction but little or no angina, the identification of dysfunctional 'hibernating' myocardium with the potential to recover following revascularization is an increasing indication for cardiac imaging. Whilst there is a large literature on the subject, there is also a great deal of confusion:

Terminology

The terms 'viable' and 'hibernating' are often used interchangeably but inappropriately. 'Viable' really refers to any area of living heart muscle, be it completely normal, myopathic, ischaemic, stunned, or hibernating. 'Hibernating' is best reserved for myocardium which is viable but dysfunctional as a result of impaired coronary flow.

Pathophysiology

'Hibernating myocardium' is a clinical concept, and the underlying pathophysiology remains controversial. At least two mechanisms are proposed:
• Reduced resting perfusion leads to downregulation of contractile function without the development of metabolic ischaemia.
• Perfusion is virtually normal at rest, but the absence of vasodilator reserve leads to demand ischaemia on minimal exertion with repetitive post-ischaemic stunning which never has the opportunity to recover.

Investigation

Every imaging modality has a way of assessing myocardial viability, but there are very few direct comparisons in the literature. It remains unclear which method or combination of methods is most appropriate and in which setting.

Rationale for treatment

Most studies have focussed on functional improvement of myocardial segments following revascularization, an end-point which is of no clinical relevance. Few have looked at improvement of overall left ventricular systolic function, let alone symptomatic or prognostic benefit.

Benefits of treatment

There is an impression that revascularization is beneficial for patients with significant hibernating myocardium, but not for those with scar. In a pooled analysis of a number of studies, patients with impaired left ventricular function and little viable myocardium were at high risk (17%) of cardiac events whether revascularized or not.[1] Those with significant viable myocardium were at similarly high risk if managed conservatively (20%), but at lower risk following revascularization (7%). However, all studies to date have been retrospective and non-randomized, and therefore vulnerable to important selection biases.

References

1 Bax JJ, van der Wall EE, Harbinson M. Radionuclide techniques for the assessment of myocardial viability and hibernation. *Heart* 2004; **90**: v26–33.

Assessment for hibernating myocardium (2)

Elements of a hibernation study

Myocardium that is likely to improve its function following revascularization should be:
- Dysfunctional at rest.
- Viable.
- Easily rendered ischaemic with stress.

A contemporary SPECT study has the potential to provide all three types of information from, respectively:
- Gated acquisition.
- Resting perfusion study.
- Stress perfusion study.

^{201}Tl and ^{99m}Tc-labelled tracers

Myocardial uptake of ^{201}Tl and ^{99m}Tc-labelled radiopharmaceuticals requires sarcolemmal integrity to maintain the electrochemical gradient, and preserved metabolic activity. In principle, uptake of tracer on a resting SPECT acquisition indicates myocardial viability, whilst its absence indicates scar.

^{201}Tl

Post-stress redistribution imaging at 4 hours significantly underestimates the amount of viability, with up to 50% of apparently fixed defects improving function with subsequent revascularization. Late redistribution imaging at 24 hours, or preferably reinjection imaging, is therefore required when a hibernation study is performed (see page 114). Uptake on any resting acquisition indicates viability in the most general sense, but *changes* in uptake between acquisitions are more specific for hibernating myocardium (e.g. stress to 4 hours redistribution, 4 hours redistribution to 24 hours redistribution, 4 hours redistribution to reinjection).

^{99m}Tc-labelled tracers

The resting injection should be performed under nitrate cover for optimal detection of viability. Whilst many experts prefer ^{201}Tl as a simple viability tracer, the ability to gate ^{99m}Tc studies to assess left ventricular function at rest, post-stress, and even with low-dose dobutamine (to assess contractile reserve as with echo) is an important advantage.

Interpretation of SPECT hibernation study

The aim of imaging is to divide patients into those with 'significant' hibernation who should be considered for revascularization, and those with 'no significant' hibernation who require conservative management. Conventionally the threshold for clinical significance is taken to be
- Tracer uptake of at least 50–60% maximum counts
- In at least 25% of the left ventricular myocardium.

In reality, the extent and transmurality of myocardial viability is a continuum, and this is reflected in the results of SPECT. The activity of ^{201}Tl or ^{99m}Tc in myocardial segments is closely related to the proportion of intact myocardium on biopsy.[1,2] Moreover, the probability of regional functional recovery following revascularization is almost linearly related to tracer uptake (Fig. 10.9).[3] A 50–60% uptake cut-off represents a level at which there is a 50% chance of functional recovery, and is therefore a pragmatic balance between positive and negative predictive accuracy. However, confidence increases with increasing distance from this threshold.

Comparison with other modalities

Few studies have directly compared the performance of different imaging modalities, each of which looks at a different aspect of myocardial viability. The preferred technique in a given centre is usually determined by availability and expertise. SPECT and dobutamine echo (for contractile reserve) are the usual 'work-horses'. The former is generally considered to have higher sensitivity (90% versus 74%), and the latter higher specificity (78% versus 57%).

Positron emission tomography ([18]FDG uptake) has traditionally been considered the optimal technique, but is expensive and not widely available (see Chapter 12). Cardiac magnetic resonance imaging (late gadolinium enhancement to delineate scar) is becoming increasingly popular, but is not widely available and outcome data is even scarcer than with the other techniques.

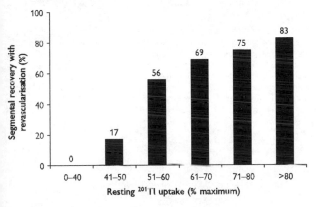

Fig. 10.9 Relationship between ^{201}Tl uptake on rest-redistribution imaging at 4 hours and probability of functional improvement with revascularization, reproduced with permission.[3]

References

1 Zimmermann R, Mall G, Rauch B, et al. Residual ^{201}Tl activity in irreversible defects as a marker of myocardial viability. Clinicopathological study. Circulation 1995; **91**: 1016–21.

2 Dakik HA, Howell JF, Lawrie GM, et al. Assessment of myocardial viability with ^{99m}Tc-sestamibi tomography before coronary bypass graft surgery: correlation with histopathology and post-operative improvement in cardiac function. Circulation 1997; **96**: 2892–8.

3 Perrone-Filardi P, Pace L, Prastaro M, et al. Assessment of myocardial viability in patients with chronic coronary artery disease. Rest-4-hour-24-hour 201Tl tomography versus dobutamine echocardiography. Circulation 1996; **94**: 2712–9.

Imaging with iodine-123-labelled radiopharmaceuticals

Iodine-123-labelled radiopharmaceuticals

Introduction

Nuclear cardiology techniques offer the potential to image aspects of myocardial physiology and metabolism which are not accessible to other imaging modalities. Positron emission tomography (PET) has been extensively used in this area, but for single photon emission computed tomography (SPECT) imaging the range of radiopharmaceuticals available is limited. Two radiopharmaceuticals labelled with iodine-123 (^{123}I) have been extensively evaluated over a number of years, though neither is yet in routine clinical use:

- ^{123}I-meta-iodo-benzyl-guanidine (^{123}I-MIBG).
- β-methyl-p-[^{123}I]iodo-phenyl-pentadecanoic acid (^{123}I-BMIPP).

The first is used to image sympathetic innervation, and the second to image fatty acid metabolism.

Physical properties of ^{123}I

- Cyclotron-generated radionuclide
- Half-life 13.3 hours.
- Decays by electron capture to ^{123}Te.
- Principal emitted photon is γ ray at 159keV.

Iodine-123-meta-iodo-benzyl-guanidine (^{123}I-MIBG)

Physiological properties of MIBG

- False neurotransmitter at sympathetic nerve endings, with similar uptake and storage to norepinephrine.
- Routinely used to image phaeochromocytomas.
- Taken up by sympathetic nerve endings in the heart via sodium- and energy-dependent 'uptake-1' mechanism.

Imaging protocol

- Thyroid blockade with potassium perchlorate 400mg orally (then 200mg 6 hourly for 24 hours).
- 30 minutes later, intravenous injection of ^{123}I-MIBG 185-370MBq.
- Early imaging at 15 minutes, with delayed imaging at 4 hours:
  - Planar acquisition in anterior projection.
  - SPECT acquisition.

Image analysis

The overall cardiac uptake of ^{123}I-MIBG can be quantified as the heart-to-mediastinum (H/M) ratio on the anterior planar projection (Fig. 11.1):

$$\frac{\text{Mean counts per pixel}_{\text{cardiac region of interest}}}{\text{Mean counts per pixel}_{\text{superior mediastinal region of interest}}}$$

The washout rate from early to delayed imaging is calculated from the following formula, which considers the radioactive decay of ^{123}I:

$$\frac{(H_1 - M_1)/(\frac{1}{2})^{t_1/T} - (H_2 - M_2)/(\frac{1}{2})^{t_2/T}}{(H_1 - M_1)/(\frac{1}{2})^{t_1/T}}$$

where H and M are the mean counts per pixel in the heart and mediastinal regions of interest (H_1 and M_1 early, H_2 and M_2 delayed), t_1 and t_2 are the times from tracer injection to early and delayed acquisition, and T is the half-life of ^{123}I (13.3 hours).

In normal individuals, the H/M ratio on the early acquisition is greater than 1.8, with a washout rate on the delayed acquisition of less than 10%. Regional denervation can be visualized on the reconstructed SPECT acquisitions.

Clinical value

Dilated cardiomyopathy

Several studies have demonstrated reduced ^{123}I-MIBG uptake with increased washout in patients with dilated cardiomyopathy. An H/M ratio <1.2 predicts adverse cardiac events independently of other factors, including left ventricular ejection fraction.[1] Whilst these findings are interesting, ^{123}I-MIBG imaging would only be of clinical importance if it could be used to guide management, perhaps in the selection of high-risk patients for an implantable defibrillator. Studies are currently underway in this area.

Coronary artery disease

Sympathetic nerve terminals are more sensitive to ischaemia than myocytes. Following myocardial infarction, the area of sympathetic denervation demonstrated by ^{123}I-MIBG SPECT is typically larger than the infarct size demonstrated using a perfusion tracer, and better reflects the initial ischaemic area at risk. Moreover, following transmural infarction, the ^{123}I-MIBG defect extends more apically than the infarct due to interruption of nerve fibres coursing apically within the epicardium. These findings are not yet of direct clinical relevance, but there is evidence that denervation of areas of viable myocardium may predispose to ventricular dysrhythmias.

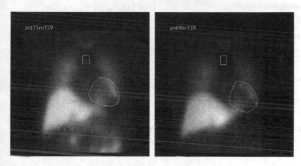

Fig. 11.1 Early and delayed anterior planar acquisitions following injection of ^{123}I-MIBG. This patient had had a left ventricular assist device explanted following recovery from severe left ventricular failure. Cardiac and mediastinal regions of interest are shown; H/M ratio was 2.6 on the early acquisition, with a washout rate of 5%, both reassuring features.

References

1 Merlet P, Benvenuti C, Moyse D, *et al.* Prognostic value of MIBG imaging in idiopathic dilated cardiomyopathy. *J Nucl Med* 1999; **40**: 917–23.

β-methyl-p-[^{123}I]iodo-phenyl-pentadecanoic acid (^{123}I-BMIPP)

Physiological properties of BMIPP

- Methyl-branched fatty acid analogue.
- Taken up by myocytes and converted to BMIPP-CoA.
- Unable to be β-oxidized, and enters intracellular lipid store.

Normal myocardium metabolizes free fatty acids in preference to glucose, but this reverses during ischaemia. Subsequently, fatty acids are directed to triglyceride synthesis rather than β-oxidation. The return to the normal state may take hours or days depending on the severity of the ischaemia. The uptake of BMIPP is therefore reduced during and after ischaemia ('ischaemic memory').

Imaging protocol

- Intravenous injection of ^{123}I-BMIPP in the fasting state.
- 30 minutes later, SPECT acquisition.

Clinical value

A number of Japanese studies have evaluated ^{123}I-BMIPP clinically, but the tracer is not readily available in Europe.

Ischaemic area at risk post reperfusion

For several days after reperfusion for myocardial infarction, the extent of the ^{123}I-BMIPP defect reflects the original ischaemic area at risk, as opposed to the more limited final infarct size.

Hibernation assessment

Myocardial segments with maintained ^{201}Tl uptake (viable) but reduced ^{123}I-BMIPP uptake (ischaemic) are likely to be hibernating.

Suspected acute coronary syndrome

^{123}I-BMIPP imaging demonstrates defects for several hours after the resolution of ischaemic chest pain, and may be more sensitive than rest perfusion imaging.

Exercise-induced ischaemia

Defects are seen following injection of ^{123}I-BMIPP at rest for several hours after exercise-induced ischaemia, mirroring exercise ^{201}Tl defects.[1] The significance of this for the routine investigation of suspected stable coronary disease remains uncertain.

References

1 Dilsizian V, Bateman TM, Bergmann SR, et al. Metabolic imaging with beta-methyl-p-[^{123}I]-iodophenylpentadecanoic acid identifies ischemic memory after demand ischemia. *Circulation* 2005; **112**: 2169–74.

Cardiac positron emission tomography (PET)

Introduction to cardiac positron emission tomography (PET)

As in single photon emission computed tomography (SPECT), positron emission tomography (PET) involves the injection of a radiopharmaceutical, the physiological properties of which determine its distribution within the patient. The labelling radionuclide then allows this distribution to be imaged. In contrast to SPECT, the positron-emitting radionuclides used in PET produce pairs of high energy 511keV γ photons travelling in opposite directions. These are not easily imaged using standard gamma camera technology, but require an alternative scintigraphic approach called coincidence detection.

The value of cardiac PET as a routine clinical tool has been limited by the expense and scarcity of cameras and the short half-lives of the radionuclides, making them difficult to handle and necessitating an on-site cyclotron and radiochemistry facilities. A number of recent developments have led to renewed interest in cardiac PET, particularly in the USA:

- Proliferation of PET/computed tomography (CT) cameras for oncology.
- Availability of commercially produced and distributed ^{18}F-fluorodeoxyglucose (^{18}F-FDG).
- Availability of perfusion tracer rubidium-82 (^{82}Rb) from generator.

For clinical purposes, cardiac PET is used in two ways:

- Stress-rest myocardial perfusion imaging, using ^{82}Rb or, now less commonly, ^{13}N-ammonia.
- Hibernation imaging, using ^{18}F-FDG to assess metabolic viability and ^{13}N-ammonia or ^{82}Rb to assess perfusion.

Cardiac PET is a specialized imaging technique, and compared with SPECT is practised in a relatively limited number of centres. The following pages are intended as an introduction only.

PET instrumentation (1)

Scintillation detectors for PET

A PET camera consists of a series of circular or hexagonal arrays of scintillation detectors, each of which is paired via a coincidence circuit with a large number of detectors on the opposite side. Multiple rings are used to improve the sensitivity of the device and acquire data from multiple cross sections simultaneously.

Sodium iodide has poor detection efficiency for high energy 511keV photons and is not a suitable scintillator for use in PET. Bismuth germanate (BGO) has been the most commonly used scintillator, but may in time be replaced by lutetium oxyorthosilicate (LSO) and/or gadolinium oxyorthosilicate (GSO). LSO and GSO have higher light production per keV of absorbed energy, and hence superior energy resolution and scatter rejection. Moreover, the phosphorent decay time is shorter, allowing better operation at high count rates.

A PET camera contains several thousand separate crystals. Instead of using the same number of separate photomultiplier tubes (PMTs), the electronic complexity and cost of the instrument is reduced by arranging the detectors in blocks coupled to a smaller number of PMTs. As with an Anger gamma camera, each detector can be identified by the pulse height distribution generated in the PMTs.

Coincidence detection

Within a short distance of the site of decay (e.g. 0.22mm for ^{18}F), an emitted positron annihilates by combining with an electron, producing two 511keV γ photons travelling in opposite directions (180° apart). If each of a pair of detectors simultaneously registers a scintillation event (coincidence), positron annihilation is assumed to have occurred along a narrow corridor between the two detectors (Fig. 12.1). In this way, coincidence detection is able to localize the site of decay within the patient without the need for collimation.

Spatial resolution and accidental coincidences

Spatial resolution in PET is determined by the area of the detectors, and is typically 5–8mm. In contrast to SPECT, the sensitivity and resolution of a pair of detectors is independent of the location of the radioactive source within the field of view.

Spatial resolution can be eroded by accidental coincidences as a result of
• Scatter coincidence, where one of the γ photons from an annihilation undergoes Compton scatter before arriving at a detector.
• Random coincidence, where γ photons from two separate but simultaneous annihilations arrive at a pair of detectors.
The problem can be reduced by minimizing the resolution time of the coincidence circuit, and using the counts from an additional accidental coincidence circuit, with a small delay between the outputs of the detector pair, to correct the counts obtained from the true coincidence circuit.

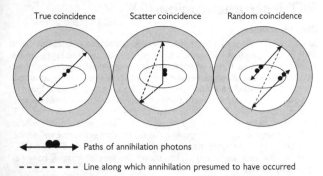

True coincidence   Scatter coincidence   Random coincidence

◀━━━●●━━━▶ Paths of annihilation photons

━ ━ ━ ━ ━ ━ ━ Line along which annihilation presumed to have occurred

Fig. 12.1 Coincidence detection. When a 511keV photon is simultaneously detected by two opposing detectors, a coincidence is registered and a positron-electron annihilation event is assumed to have occurred along a line between the detectors. In addition to true coincidences, scatter coincidences and random coincidences also occur, eroding spatial resolution.

PET instrumentation (2)

Photon scatter

BGO has relatively poor energy resolution, so scatter is a potential problem with BGO-dependent PET cameras. To reduce scatter, lead septa can be placed between each ring of detectors to ensure that only coincidences from detectors in the same ring or a few adjacent rings will be admitted: 'septa-in' or 'two-dimensional' mode. The lead septa provide a form of collimation and reduce the sensitivity of the system, but to a much lesser extent than in SPECT. Development of the latest generation of PET cameras is being driven by the need to increase sensitivity for whole body oncology imaging by removing the septa: 'three-dimensional' mode. This has been made more practical by the introduction of LSO and GSO crystals. The advantages and disadvantages for cardiac imaging have yet to be fully defined.

Attenuation correction and reconstruction

Attenuation is a bigger problem in PET than in SPECT: although the two 511keV photons resulting from positron annihilation each have a relatively low attenuation coefficient, both must reach a detector for a coincidence to be registered. Attenuation correction is therefore essential in PET, but is easier and more accurate than in SPECT as the length of the path of attenuation is constant and known (the distance between any two detectors). A rotating line source (germanium-68 or cesium-137) or X-ray CT is used to assess attenuation through different parts of the patient, and this is used to correct the true coincidences. The corrected data are then used to reconstruct the image using filtered back projection. X-ray CT offers a high-resolution transmission map in less than a minute, but care must be taken to avoid and recognize misregistration with the emission scan, a prime cause of artefacts.

Gamma camera imaging of positron-emitting tracers

Attempts have been made to image positron-emitting radiopharmaceuticals (usually ^{18}F-FDG) on a gamma camera, in order to make these tracers more relevant in everyday nuclear medicine. This can be done using SPECT imaging with a thick sodium iodide crystal and heavy high-energy collimators, but the sensitivity is poor compared with PET or ^{99m}Tc SPECT. Alternatively, a dual-headed camera with the detectors uncollimated and positioned 180° apart can be used to perform coincidence detection. Such systems are significantly inferior to dedicated PET cameras, and most manufacturers are not currently pursuing their development.

Radiopharmaceuticals for cardiac PET (1)

Introduction

Radionuclides used in gamma camera imaging are not isotopes of the biochemically relevant elements carbon, hydrogen, oxygen and nitrogen, so the physiological and metabolic information they can provide is limited. The only γ-emitting isotopes of carbon, oxygen, and nitrogen that can be used for imaging are positron-emitters (^{11}C, ^{15}O, ^{13}N), whilst fluorine-18 (^{18}F) can be used to substitute for −OH in a number of metabolically relevant molecules. These radionuclides have relatively short half-lives, so the requirement for an on-site cyclotron and radiochemistry facilities has restricted the value of cardiac PET as a routine clinical tool.

Two important developments have generated renewed interest in cardiac PET, particularly in the USA:
• Availability of commercially produced and distributed ^{18}F-FDG, primarily to supply the oncology market.
• Availability of ^{82}Rb generators, allowing perfusion imaging.

The most commonly used cardiac PET radiopharmaceuticals are ^{13}N-ammonia, ^{82}Rb and ^{18}F-FDG, and are described below. ^{15}O-H$_2$O is an ideal perfusion tracer with an extraction fraction of 100%, and provides excellent absolute flow quantification for research applications. However it is not used for imaging and will not be considered further.

^{13}N-ammonia

Physical and physiological properties
• Longstanding PET perfusion tracer.
• Only used in centres with on-site cyclotron.
• ^{13}N decays by positron emission to stable ^{13}C, with half-life 10 minutes.
• Excellent first pass extraction fraction (95%).
• Passive diffusion into myocytes, with adenosine triphosphate (ATP)-dependent retention as ^{13}N-glutamine.

Protocol
• Inject 370–740MBq intravenously.
• Commence acquisition after 1.5–3.0 minutes for 5–15 minutes.
• Perform at rest, and repeat with pharmacological stress after 40 minutes (if full perfusion study required).

Radiopharmaceuticals for cardiac PET (2)

^{82}Rb

Physical and physiological properties

- Available from commercially produced generator; replaced every 4 weeks.
- Parent radionuclide strontium-82 (^{82}Sr) decays to ^{82}Rb by electron capture, with half-life 25.5 days.
- ^{82}Rb decays by positron emission to stable ^{82}Kr, with half-life 75 seconds.
- ^{82}Rb eluted with saline as required using computer-controlled pump connected to intravenous cannula in patient; repeat imaging can be performed after 5 minutes, when 90% maximal available activity present.
- ^{82}Rb is monovalent cation with extraction fraction similar to ^{201}Tl.

Protocol

- Scout scan for positioning (small dose ^{82}Rb or CT).
- Inject 1480–2220MBq intravenously (typical dose for 'two-dimensional' mode with BGO-based camera).
- Commence acquisition after 70–90 seconds (if normal left ventricular function) for 3–6 minutes.
- Perform at rest, and repeat with pharmacological stress after 10–15 minutes.
- Complete study can be performed in a little over 30 minutes in experienced centres.

^{18}F-FDG

Physical and physiological properties

- Widely used PET metabolic tracer; used in cardiac imaging to demonstrate myocardial viability or 'ischaemic memory'.
- Relatively long half-life of ^{18}F allows ^{18}F-FDG to be commercially produced and distributed, without the need for an on-site cyclotron.
- ^{18}F decays by positron emission to stable ^{18}O, with half-life 110 minutes.
- ^{18}F-FDG is a glucose analogue which enters myocytes via GLUT4 transporter.
- Phosphorylated intracellularly to ^{18}F-FDG-phosphate which is a poor substrate for further metabolism and accumulates in proportion to glycolytic rate of cell.

Protocol

In the fasting state, the myocardium preferentially metabolizes free fatty acids. In the fed state, the increase in plasma glucose leads to insulin secretion, inhibiting fatty acid release and increasing myocardial glucose uptake and utilization. ^{18}F-FDG imaging must therefore be performed in the presence of insulin. In a non-diabetic, this is best achieved by giving an oral glucose load to stimulate endogenous insulin secretion. Supplementary intravenous doses of insulin are frequently required to achieve an optimal blood glucose level of 5.6–7.8mmol/l at the time of ^{18}F FDG injection. Diabetics are a particular problem and a number of protocols are available which use some combination of intravenous glucose and insulin.

- Inject 185–555MBq intravenously.
- Commence acquisition after 45–60 minutes for 10–30 minutes.

Interpretation and clinical significance of cardiac PET studies

Perfusion imaging with ¹³N-ammonia or ⁸²Rb

Reconstructed and reorientated stress and rest slices are displayed according to the same conventions as SPECT. Interpretation is similar to SPECT, but images are usually of superior quality and free of attenuation. This permits greater confidence in reporting, with higher diagnostic accuracy.[1]

There is accumulating evidence of the prognostic value of ⁸²Rb PET perfusion imaging.[2]

It is unlikely that PET will replace SPECT as the 'work horse' for radionuclide myocardial perfusion imaging, but it may find a role in the investigation of specific groups of patients in enthusiastic centres (e.g. those with a previous equivocal SPECT study, or who are likely to have marked soft tissue attenuation).

Hibernation and ischaemia assessment with ¹⁸F-FDG

Reconstructed and reorientated ¹⁸F-FDG slices are displayed alongside rest (and, if available, stress) perfusion slices (using ¹³N-ammonia or ⁸²Rb) according to the same conventions as SPECT. Pixels in the ¹⁸F-FDG slices are normalized to the maximal counts in the rest perfusion study.

Myocardial hibernation

PET ¹⁸F-FDG imaging is usually considered to be the most sensitive form of imaging for identifying hibernating myocardium. Dysfunctional myocardial segments with
- Preserved ¹⁸F-FDG uptake despite reduced resting perfusion (perfusion-metabolism mismatch) are hibernating and likely to recover function following revascularization.
- Reduced ¹⁸F-FDG uptake in proportion to reduced resting perfusion are scar and unlikely to recover function following revascularization.

In one study, the presence of hibernating myocardium amounting to 30% or more of the myocardium predicted improvement in overall left ventricular systolic function following revascularization with sensitivity 86% and specificity 92% (Fig. 12.2).[3]

'Ischaemic memory' imaging

Ischaemic myocardium ceases to metabolize free fatty acids, and depends instead on glucose metabolism to generate high-energy phosphates via glycolysis. This state persists for several hours after the resolution of ischaemia. It has been proposed that ¹⁸F-FDG PET be use as an investigation in acute chest pain to identify previously ischaemic myocardium. Such 'hot spot' metabolic imaging is performed together with rest perfusion imaging to provide a myocardial 'road map'.

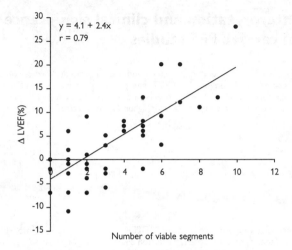

Fig. 12.2 Improvement in global left ventricular ejection fraction following revascularization as a function of the number of viable myocardial segments according to ^{18}F-FDG, reproduced with permission.[3]

References

1 Bateman TM, Heller GV, McGhie AI, et al. Diagnostic accuracy of rest/stress ECG-gated Rb-82 myocardial perfusion PET: comparison with ECG-gated Tc-99m sestamibi SPECT. *J Nucl Cardiol* 2006; **13**: 24–33.

2 Yoshinaga K, Chow BJW, Williams K, et al. What is the prognostic value of myocardial perfusion imaging using rubidium-82 positron emission tomography? *J Am Coll Cardiol* 2006; **48**: 1029–39.

3 Bax JJ, Visser FC, Poldermans D, et al. Relationship between preoperative viability and postoperative improvement in LVEF and heart failure symptoms. *J Nucl Med* 2001; **42**: 79–86.

Index